# A SQUARE MEAL

# A Square Meal

## A CULINARY HISTORY OF
## THE GREAT DEPRESSION

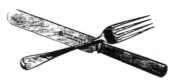

## Jane Ziegelman

### AND

## Andrew Coe

HARPER

*An Imprint of* HarperCollins*Publishers*

HarperCollins books may be purchased for educational, business, or sales promotional use. For information, please e-mail the Special Markets Department at SPsales@harpercollins.com.

FIRST EDITION

*Designed by Fritz Metsch*

Library of Congress Cataloging-in-Publication Data

Ziegelman, Jane, and Coe, Andrew
A square meal : a culinary history of the Great Depression / Jane Ziegelman and Andrew Coe.
p.   cm
Includes bibliographical references and index.
ISBN: 978-0-06-221641-0

1. Cooking, American—History—20th century. 2. Depressions—1929—United States. 3. Crises—United States—History—20th century. 4. Social change—United States—History—20th century. 5. Food supply—United States—History—20th century. 6. Diet—United States—History—20th century. 7. Home economics—United States—History—20th century. 8. Cooking—History. 9. United States—Social conditions—1933–1945. 10. United States—Environmental conditions—History—20th century.

TX715.Z54   2016
641.597309/04                                            2016016051

16 17 18 19 20   OV/RRD   10 9 8 7 6 5 4 3 2 1

*To Buster and Edward*

# Acknowledgments

T HE RESEARCH AND writing of this book spanned a huge
variety of topics, from public policy to hobo lore, and
took us on a journey through historical documents to
every corner of the United States. We could not have completed
it without considerable help from numerous libraries, archives,
and individuals. Home base for our research was the New York
Public Library's General Research Division, but we also relied
on important collections in New York University's Bobst Library,
particularly the Fales Library's Marion Nestle Food Studies Collection, the Rare Book & Manuscript Library at Columbia University's Butler Library, and the Library of Congress. The Special
Collections division of the Cornell University Library generously
provided access to archives of the school's Department of Home
Economics, including important correspondence with Eleanor
Roosevelt. For research into the policy and politics of food and
relief, we relied on the vast resources of the National Archives and
Records Administration, including its College Park, Maryland,
facility; Kansas City, Missouri, division (for the Bureau of Home
Economics records); Herbert Hoover Presidential Library; and,
most important, the Franklin D. Roosevelt Presidential Library in
Hyde Park, New York. The friendly and exceedingly helpful staff
of the National Agricultural Library helped us retrieve a trove of
material related to the United States Department of Agriculture

and its Bureau of Home Economics. Other libraries that gave us crucial research assistance were the Bentley Historical Library at the University of Michigan and the California State Library, whose Emily Blodget was a huge help. Among the many experts who gave us research guidance and material were Eleanor Arnold, Carole Eberly, and especially Anne Mendelson for her wise counsel and her *America Eats!* files. The Writers' Studio at the New York Mercantile Library has been a welcome haven for writing and contemplating our next meal. We would like to thank our agent, Jason Yarn, who was always ready to leap into the breach when we needed a hand (and an extension), and, of course, our very patient editor, Bill Strachan, who stood by us during the too many years it took to complete this book. We endured the effort thanks in part to the friendship and support of the Weekend Flushing Eats Crew, who kept up our spirits with the help of copious amounts of good food.

# Contents

*A  SQUARE  MEAL*

# *Prologue*

———•◦•———

ARLY ON THE morning of November 11, 1918, on a railroad car in northern France, a German delegation signed the Armistice agreement, signaling the end of hostilities and the complete defeat of the German army, to go into effect at 11 a.m. that day. At 10:59 a.m., the last soldier was killed in World War I: an American infantryman from Baltimore named Henry Gunther, who ignored orders and senselessly charged a pair of German machine guns. When the hour was reached, the guns grew silent on the fields of battle that stretched across the western front. For the 1.2 million troops of the American Expeditionary Force, the Armistice ended the largest and bloodiest battle in American history, the Meuse-Argonne Offensive, in which 26,000 U.S. soldiers had been killed. The survivors were exhausted and often shell-shocked, suffering from trench foot, fleas, lice, scabies, dysentery, and a host of other ailments. They packed their mess kits, blankets, trench tools, gas masks, and other gear in their field packs, shouldered their rifles, and began their march to the railway lines, where they would begin their journeys home. Despite the privations they had undergone, the Americans held one great advantage over both the German enemy and the soldiers of their French and British allies. They were by far the best-fed troops of World War I.

The U.S. Army field ration in France varied according to circumstances, but the core of the soldiers' daily diet was twenty ounces of fresh beef (or sixteen ounces of canned meat or twelve ounces of bacon), twenty ounces of potatoes, and eighteen ounces of bread, hard or soft. American troops were always proud that they enjoyed white bread, while all the other armies had to subsist on dark breads of various sorts. This ration was supplemented with coffee, sugar, salt, pepper, dried fruit, and jam. If supply lines were running, a soldier could eat almost four pounds of food, or 5,000 calories, a day. American generals believed that this was the best diet for building bone, muscle, tissue, and endurance. British and French troops consumed closer to 4,000 calories, while in the last months of the war the Germans were barely receiving enough rations to sustain themselves. Compared to noncombatants, they were relatively lucky. Across the war zones of Belgium, northern France, and eastern Europe, many thousands of women, children, and old people had starved to death. Away from the front lines strict rationing was the rule, with barely any meat available to civilians. In the history of Europe this hunger was nothing new, just the latest in the series of famines that had swept across the continent over the centuries.

The U.S. Army owed its stupendous culinary fortune to the richness of the American soil, the hard work of its farmers, and a man named Herbert Hoover. Shortly after the United States entered the war in April 1917, President Wilson asked Hoover, a brilliant mining engineer who was then directing food relief to Belgium, to reorganize the American food system to support the war effort. Operating under the slogan of "Food Will Win the War," the U.S. Food Administration sold farmers fertilizer at discount prices and encouraged them to expand their acreage and adopt the latest scientific farming practices. Hoover also fixed agricultural prices to avoid inflation and took control of railway lines to ensure rapid shipment of foodstuffs to East Coast ports, where ships were loaded with Maine potatoes, beef and pork from the Chicago stockyards, Dakota wheat, and dried fruits from Oregon and California. If the merchant fleets were able to avoid German U-boats, the food would arrive in Europe to be distributed to Allied troops, hungry refugees in Belgium and northern France, mess halls, field kitchens, and frontline trenches.

During the war, the troops' unofficial motto had been "Heaven, Hell, or Hoboken by Christmas." Most had embarked for Europe from the Hoboken docks; if they survived the conflict, they hoped to land again at Hoboken. In reality, the majority of them missed Christmas, at least in 1918, and the ships carrying them home also landed at Boston, Newport News, and Charleston. For the returning, often seasick troops, their first view of American soil somehow seemed to take place early in the morning, in the fog. Nevertheless, their greeting back in American waters—even before they landed—was rapturous. Local governments, newspapers, and anybody else who could chartered boats to race out to meet the arriving ships. When the *Mauretania*, carrying 3,999 troops, steamed into New York Harbor late in 1918, a police boat carrying the mayor's welcoming committee pulled alongside. After city dignitaries shouted greetings to them through megaphones, the troops who crowded the deck and hung from every porthole bellowed en masse: "When do we eat?!"[1] It became a custom for greeting parties to hire professional baseball pitchers to hurl California oranges at the troops—some soldiers sustained concussions from the barrage—to give them their first taste of fresh American produce in more than a year, a prelude to the series of memorable feasts that would mark the rest of their journeys home.

After the boats tied up, teams of young women from local Red Cross canteens rushed on board with coffee, sandwiches, and doughnuts to distribute to the soldiers. The next order of business was a homecoming parade, more than five hundred of which were held in cities across the country. The biggest parades were staged in New York City, where Fifth Avenue from the Washington Square Arch north was festooned with lanterns and American flags. At almost every parade, crowds threw gifts of fruit and candy to the passing troops. In Boston,

> *groups of enthusiasts at various points along the route did their best to regale the marching men with fruit, candy and sandwiches. In some places, these things were tossed from windows just above street level, and, in spite of the best efforts of the soldiers fell smashing upon the pavement, until the street at such points was littered with samples of various kinds of goodies, from chocolates and bonbons, through the small catalogues of package goods to oranges and bananas.*[2]

Traveling in open cars and holding bouquets of welcome, the wounded were also pelted: "Their laps were piled high with oranges and sandwiches, and many had bottles of lemon pop, in the enjoyment of which it appeared that flowers were a hindrance."[3] The end of the parade was usually marked by a banquet, formal or informal. To honor the 26,000 troops of the 27th Division, the big New York City hotels offered them the following menu:

> *Olives. Mixed Sweet Pickles.*
> *Grape Fruit.*
> *Fresh Vegetable Soup.*
> *Half Roast Broiler.*
> *Boiled Sweet Potato. Green Peas.*
> *Apple Pie.*
> *Neapolitan Ice Cream.*
> *Large Coffee with Milk and Sugar.*
> *Bread and Butter.*
> *Cigarettes. White Rock.*[4]

In Newport News, the troops of Maryland's 115th Infantry were given a feast of "real Maryland" food, including 4,000 pounds of fried chicken, 1,800 soft-shell crabs, crab cakes, ham, biscuits, peas, asparagus, potatoes, oranges, and strawberries, all served by "two dozen of Maryland's pretty girls."[5] For soldiers whose homes were farther inland, banquets would have to wait for weeks or even months before they were finally released from military duty. Although less elaborate, these homecoming celebrations were no less enthusiastic. In Lincoln, Illinois, twenty thousand citizens gathered in mid-August heat to commemorate their heroes' return with a parade and picnic featuring fried chicken, veal loaf, potato salad, coleslaw, baked beans, pie, cake, and sandwiches.

For veterans, of course, their final and most anticipated celebration was their first home-cooked dinner. Many had been fantasizing about this for months, dreaming of such all-American specialties as chicken and dumplings, apple pie, and coffee with real cream. In reality, these homecomings could be difficult. Veterans had been strongly affected by the war—many had continuing physical and mental problems—and saw that their relatives were complacent and uninterested in their experiences. In John Dos Passos's novel *The Big Money* (the third book in his U.S.A. trilogy), veteran Charley Anderson is made uncomfortable by his family's effusive welcome at the St. Paul, Minnesota, train station. After returning home, the first order of business is a feast:

> *They had a big dinner ready and Jim gave him a drink of whiskey and old man Vogel kept pouring him out beer and saying, "Now tell us all about it." Charley sat there with his face all red, eating stewed chicken and the dumplings and drinking the beer till he was ready to burst. He couldn't think what to tell them so he made funny cracks when they asked him questions. After dinner old man Vogel gave him one of his best Havana cigars.*[6]

After a few months of restlessness and conflict with his family, Charley buys a ticket for a sleeping car berth on the New York train:

*When he woke up in the morning in the lower berth he pushed up the shade and looked out; the train was going through the Pennsylvania hills, the fields were freshplowed, some of the trees had a little fuzz of green on them. In a farmyard a flock of yellow chickens were picking around under a peartree in bloom. "By God," he said aloud, "I'm through with the sticks."*[7]

# Chapter 1

———⁕———

**T**HE FIRST SIGN of trouble was the exodus of young folk, the steady march of rural sons and daughters leaving the countryside for more promising futures in the Big City. The migration began in the years leading up to World War I and picked up speed after 1914 as farm-raised offspring flocked to high-paying jobs in urban shipyards and munitions factories. Once the fighting ended, returning soldiers—many of them country boys who had tasted the largeness of the world—now saw the farm as a jail sentence. Some never returned, depriving the farmer of his best workers, his unpaid children. The farmer's predicament found its way into the 1919 vaudeville hit "How 'Ya Gonna Keep 'Em Down on the Farm (After They've Seen Paree?)":

> *How 'ya gonna keep 'em away from Broadway,*
> *Jazzin' aroun' and paintin' the town?*
> *How 'ya gonna keep 'em away from harm? That's a mystery.*
> *They'll never want to see a rake or a plow,*
> *And who the deuce can parley-vous a cow?*
> *How 'ya gonna keep 'em down on the farm*
> *After they've seen Paree?*

The jaunty melody belied the seriousness of the question. For many anxious Americans, "city drift" was a symptom of deeper distress. Despite the goodness of the land and the many virtues of farm living, something was wrong in the American countryside.

The "rural problem," it turns out, proved a fertile ground for thought, launching a quarter century of national soul-searching. Through the second half of the nineteenth century, Progressive Era reformers like Jacob Riis and Jane Addams had focused their energies on those social evils born of the modern metropolis. The two items at the top of their agenda, the abuses of the sweatshop system and the dire living conditions found in the tenements, were strictly urban maladies. It now appeared that the countryside was also in need of reform. Like Thomas Jefferson before him, President Theodore Roosevelt saw the American farmer as the beating heart of the nation's moral, political, and spiritual life. The decline of farm life, if it continued apace, threatened both the soul of the republic and the country's ability to feed itself. In 1908, Roosevelt appointed the Country Life Commission to investigate "the failure of country life, as it exists at present, to satisfy the higher social and intellectual aspirations of country people."[1] After six months of research, the commission's report confirmed what many already suspected: a hobbling malaise had descended over rural America. As to the source of the problem, experts determined it was none other than the farmer himself. In short, the agricultural class was stuck somewhere in the nineteenth century, prisoner to its own outmoded habits and attitudes. Discussion of the rural problem was taken up by reform-minded church leaders, government bureaucrats, charity workers, and farmers themselves. It even gave rise to its own branch of social science, "rural sociology," whose practitioners studied everything that had gone wrong with country life with an eye toward fixing it. Naturally each group came to the table with its own self-interested point of view. Even so, all seemed to agree that America had essentially divided into City and Farm, two separate and largely hostile "civilizations."

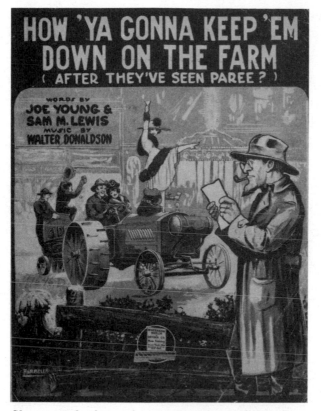

*Sheet music for the popular 1919 song memorializing the city-bound migration of rural offspring following World War I.* (Library of Congress, Notated Music Collection, 2013562671)

Since the end of the Civil War, the nation's cities had enjoyed a period of explosive growth. Factory smokestacks, the minarets of urban America, shot up along waterfronts, while rows of redbrick tenements, housing for the new industrial workforce, sprouted in their shadows. Everyday life in the modern city was defined by the surging intensity of the street, the great shopping boulevards packed with hungry consumers. The cosmopolitan mixing of class and ethnicity, a basic condition of city living, offered daily lessons in sophistication, while city saloons, cafés, theaters, and concert halls promised nonstop amusement. The hallmarks of country living, meanwhile, were isolation and self-reliance. Whatever diversions were enjoyed by country folk were home-spun affairs: box picnics at the local schoolhouse, at-home dances with the neighbors, Sunday dinners with the pastor. The baubles and smart getups so admired by urban fashion plates were un-known to rural women who sewed their own clothes, their shop-ping needs met by the Sears, Roebuck & Company catalog. The advances in technology that were revolutionizing city life had largely bypassed the farm. Deep into the 1920s, countrywomen still hauled their water from outdoor wells, cooked on wood-burning stoves, and lit their homes with kerosene. The family conveyance was most likely still a horse-drawn buggy. In the fields, a team of horses pulled the farmer's plow. Interested ob-servers seized on these differences and used them as tangible ex-amples of the growing rift. A more elusive distinction, however, involved the experience of time.

In the great urban centers, the pulse of the factory served as a kind of metronome for the city at large. In the urban workplace, where wages were paid by the hour, efficiency was a measure of success. Factory hands demonstrated their worth by completing the maximum number of standardized motions in a given period. After the factory whistle blew, their time was their own. But even at leisure, city dwellers saw time as a resource, like coal or copper. The fear that time might run out, as every resource will, left them with the dread of time wasted. On the farm, meanwhile, time was not something you stockpiled like firewood. Farm chores took as long as they took—there was no rushing an ear of corn—and the workday stretched to accommodate the tasks at hand. Time was elastic. The minutes and hours that mattered so much to city folk were irrelevant to the drawn-out biological processes on which the farmer depended. In place of the clock, the farmer's yardstick for measuring time was the progress of the seasons. As a result, his view of time was expansive, focused on the sweeping cycles of the natural world. For city people, time was fractured into finite segments like boxes on a conveyer belt. On the farm, time was continuous, like a string around a tree, one season flowing inevitably into the next.

For all their abstraction, conflicting ideas about time found concrete expression in the realm of food. Played out daily in American kitchens, culinary tensions began with the kitchen itself, a focus of enduring concern among rural reformers. To the city observer, the most striking feature of the farmhouse kitchen was its unwieldy size. In the second half of the nineteenth century, when it came time to put up a house, farmers turned for guidance to floor plans printed in agricultural journals and design manuals like Lewis Allen's 1852 *Rural Architecture*. The kitchen, as envisioned by Allen, was far and away the largest room in the house, a reflection of the many uses it served. Aside from cooking, "the chief living room," as Allen called it, doubled as the homemaker's all-purpose workshop, dining room, nursery, and, occasionally, sleeping quarters. Over the following decade, farmhouses sprouted separate dining rooms and "sitting rooms," and as a result kitchens began to shrink. When the shrinking leveled off, however, kitchens were still spacious enough to accommodate a family-size table (and families could be large), stove, sink, wood bin, floor-to-ceiling cupboard, and rocking chair.

Country reformers shuddered at all that gratuitous floor space. With so much ground to cover, the rural homemaker was condemned to walk miles each day just to prepare family meals. Those steps became the focus of scientific management, a new field founded on the ideas of men like Frederick W. Taylor. A mechanical engineer, Taylor believed that American prosperity was endangered by the "awkward, ill-directed, or inefficient movements of men." Armed with a stopwatch, he analyzed work processes in order to find the "one best way" to complete a given task in the shortest amount of time. Meanwhile, the industrial engineers Frank and Lillian Gilbreth pioneered the motion study. Using movie cameras to analyze the worker at his task, they isolated minute gestures, eliminating any that were wasteful. Lured by the promise of increased productivity, factory and office managers embraced what came to be called "time and motion" studies. Though conceived for the workplace, these studies were embraced by Progressive-minded women—mostly urban, highly educated, and well-off—who applied them to the home. Between 1910 and 1930, a flood of books and articles on household efficiency taught homemakers how to save time by standardizing daily tasks and eliminating unnecessary motions. It was found, for example, that boiling an egg could be reduced from a bloated twenty-seven motions to the more svelte fifteen. Newspaper columns urged women to put themselves on housework schedules, replacing the usual ad hoc approach to cooking and cleaning with more strategic and businesslike tactics. Predictably, domestic efficiency experts were enthusiastic spokeswomen for the new generation of household appliances targeted at the homemaker, a message echoed in the advertisements for vacuum cleaners and electric irons that filled women's magazines and promised to slash her workday.

Picking up on the efficiency craze, rural reformers directed the techniques of scientific management toward the traditional American farmhouse, with a special focus on the kitchen. Magazines from *Ladies' Home Journal* to *Threshermen's Review* published plans for more efficient kitchens, while the Department of Agriculture issued pamphlets like "The Farm Kitchen as a Workshop," proposing that rural women replace the large, multipurpose space with a compact, well-organized room used exclusively for cooking. To quantify what they already knew, in the early

1920s researchers from the Department of Agriculture equipped rural homemakers with pedometers, devices pinned to the women's aprons or strapped to their ankles that counted their steps as they went about their chores. Among their findings was that one Montana woman walked a quarter of a mile in the course of baking a lemon pie! In a second variation on the time and motion theme, government investigators asked almost two thousand farm women to keep time diaries, running accounts of time expended over twenty-four-hour periods. The women recorded their daily round of activities on circular clock charts, each circle sliced like a pie into five-minute segments. Subjects noted how much time was given to house cleaning, to laundry and sewing, to family, and so on. To no one's surprise, the charts showed that farm women devoted the lion's share of their workday to food preparation.

On the farm, the one advance women longed for most was running water, an end to all that bucket hauling. The reformers, however, saw no reason to stop at the kitchen sink. With characteristic optimism, they believed that modernity—with all its rewards—was within the women's grasp. Their mission was to empower farm women with the knowledge of what was possible, including smaller kitchens and improved kitchen habits. The main objects of their passion, however, were reserved for new labor-saving devices like gas stoves and electric dishwashers, which they declared indispensable to kitchen efficiency and urged on farm women everywhere. But change came slowly to rural America. Frustrated, reformers blamed the women for what they saw as a failure of vision. In an article promoting "step-saving" kitchens, one Iowa home economist lamented: "Many times the homemaker deprives herself of conveniences and the home of possible improvements because she waits for someone else to suggest their addition."[2] Other rural observers saw farm women

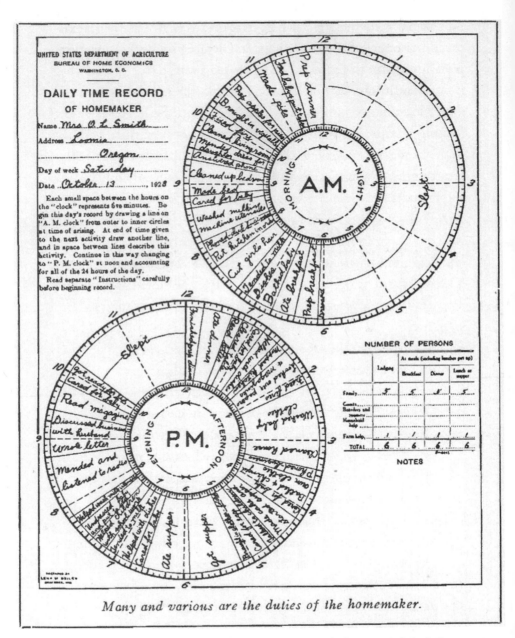

*Many and various are the duties of the homemaker.*

*As the subjects of time-use studies, farm women were asked to record their daily activities on clock charts. The woman represented here worked a sixteen-hour day.* (Maud Wilson, "The Use of Time by Oregon Home Makers," Agricultural Experiment Station, Oregon State Agricultural College, Corvallis, 1929, 41)

more harshly, depicting them as resigned to their backward existence, prisoners of their own inertia. City newspapers ran features
on the plight of the rural woman, her long workday, and primitive
living conditions. One story in the *Boston Herald* titled "The Wife
of the Farmer—The Woman God Forgot" described her with the
following adjectives: "faded and work weary . . . hidden away in
the remote corners, isolated, drudging, and alone."[3]

Country homemakers who encountered these pitiful beings in
the popular press were outraged and made their feelings known.
A Massachusetts woman named Adeline O. Goessling, an editor
at *Farm and Home,* asked subscribers what they thought of the
*Boston Herald* story and other, similar reports. In an attempt to
set the record straight, close to ten thousand women responded,
including this one from Illinois:

> *Lonely? Where is there such an abundance of life as in the
> country? There may not be crowds of people but nature makes
> a grander showing. The trees, the grass, the flowers, the birds,
> the horses and cattle—even the crickets, locusts, katydids, and
> frogs, all add to the grand symphony of nature. . . . Where
> are the members of the family nearer and dearer to each other
> than on the farm? Where do they understand each other
> better? How many wonderful evenings are spent together
> with neighbors around the piano and victrola, singing and
> dancing! How many pleasant hours are spent driving through
> the country, going to band-concerts or picnics or to church on
> Sunday! And then there are the telephones and the daily visits
> of the letter-carrier with magazines and newspapers. . . . It
> is city life that is lonely, where one may travel all day through
> crowded streets and be among strangers.*[4]

Despite her lack of modern conveniences, the farm woman, it
seems, was not so bereft as some imagined.

Satisfaction with their lot, however, did not mean that farm life was easy. In truth, countrywomen worked even harder and longer than the studies suggested. Regardless of what the clock charts indicated, the woman's role in feeding her family extended well beyond the 13.2 hours, as one study had it, spent each week in meal preparation. Through the 1920s, family farms were still largely self-sustaining. Roughly once a week, the homemaker made the trip to town to buy provisions at the general store. Her shopping list was brief: salt, coffee, sugar, baking soda, flour (if she didn't grow her own wheat), and maybe a can of salmon, a luxury food reserved for Sunday supper. In place of cash, she paid for these items with eggs from her chickens, butter from her cows, or some other farm-produced food. The bulk of her larder came straight from the land and livestock, though seldom in edible form. Before it landed on the table, farm-raised food required processing of one kind or another, a responsibility that generally fell to the homemaker. Milk needed to be strained, and butter required churning. Corn was ground into meal, and chickens were dressed. Fruits and vegetables from the woman's own garden were canned, dried, or pickled. Sorghum was stripped and crushed, the raw juice boiled down into "molasses." Apples from the family orchard were pressed into cider, which in turn was left to ferment, the homemaker's source of vinegar.

Living off the land meant that farm women experienced every phase in the chain of events that brought food to table, from planting seeds and raising chicks right up to cooking for the family. Dinnertime, the culmination of labor spread over days, weeks, or even months, was an occasion to think back on all the hard work behind them. Here, the Michigan writer Della Lutes describes the content of her mealtime musings:

> *October days ushered in the cider season and the making of apple butter. Gathering windfalls and seconds into the wagon*

*to be taken to the mill was another of those homely tasks that
gave zest to the lives of country folk, for here again you reaped
the fruits of your own labor, as when, for instance, you carried
your own meal home for your own johnnycake. When you ate
buckwheat cakes in winter you thought of that hot July Fourth
when it had been sown, "wet or dry." You smelled the bee-sweet
odor of small white orchid–like flowers upheld on their stout,
wine-colored stems and heard the hum of a million wings. . . .
Like God, you looked back upon your work and called it good.[5]*

This woman, who audaciously compared herself to the "Heavenly
Father," would have never imagined that she was guilty of ineffi-
ciency.

Rural women were not averse to technology. On the contrary,
they saw the benefits of electrified homes and, above all, running
water, not to mention the paved roads that would help remedy
the problem of rural isolation. At the same time, however, they
exulted in the unique satisfactions that came from living off the
land. As a woman of letters, Della Lutes was particularly eloquent
on the topic, but thousands of women expressed similar feelings.
A woman's ability to coax food from the soil filled her with an
appreciation for her own usefulness. For one midwestern homemaker who participated in a 1924 government survey, the generosity of the soil was an ongoing source of wonderment:

*You don't think of your home on a farm as just a space in-
side four walls. The feeling of home spreads out all around,
into the garden, the orchards, the henhouses, the barn, the
springhouse, because you are all the time helping to produce
live things in those places and they or their products, are all
the time coming back into your kitchen from garden, orchard,
barn or henhouse, as part of the things you handle and prepare for meals or market every day.*

The country homemaker was endlessly moving between her kitchen and the natural world to the point where the two were merged, "one of the peculiarities," the woman points out, "of making a home on the farm."[6] These were the very same "peculiarities" that the time-use studies were essentially designed to ignore. Counting the number of minutes spent in one "division of work" or another, categories devised by the investigators, obscured the fluid nature of farmhouse living. Chores did not begin and end in the way depicted on the clock charts.

Efficiency experts took it on faith that old-fashioned housework was the homemaker's burden. Her fulfillment, they reasoned, was found in leisure time when she could cultivate the "higher life" through reading and attending women's clubs and church socials. Farm women, conversely, understood that "honest" work was a satisfaction in its own right: "I have lived on a farm more than forty years . . . and my back is straight as a dart yet. Worked any? Yes, indeed, at a good stiff pace and why not? The world's work must be done and I am no shirk."[7] Of their daily tasks, none offered the same satisfactions as cooking for the family. A woman's standing in the community rested partly on her culinary skills. For farm women, the pleasures of cooking were their own reward:

> *They delight greatly in their beautiful well-filled cellars with an esthetic as well as a gastronomic joy. They speak so feelingly of sweet juicy hams and new-laid eggs, golden butter and batches of white bread, apple pies, berry pies, pumpkin pies, barrels of sparkling cider, fresh crisp vegetables, rich ice cream, luscious watermelons and peaches, pungent mincemeat, and crunchy spiced pickles that the reader is almost consumed with hunger—and envy. It is the supreme satisfaction of the country woman to thus look upon her work for the family and find it good, and*

*to know that whatever happens during the long winter, her dear ones will not suffer from hunger.*[8]

These testimonies from farm women, however, did not register with many home economists and others overseeing rural studies. In fact, when researchers found evidence that farm women were satisfied with their lives, they frequently found cause to dismiss it and deliberately omitted testimonials from contented home-makers.

In the welter of time-use studies focused on rural cooks, one topic received little attention. The food these women labored over was immaterial to the efficiency calculus, and home economists saw no reason to clutter their reports with culinary specifics. They were fully attentive, however, to nutritional issues, another subject of intensive research. The gold standard of rural dietary studies was a 1923 survey of 1,331 families in the Farm Belt states of Kansas, Kentucky, Missouri, and Ohio that showed that the average farmhouse diet made liberal use of just about every food group. For example, Kansas and Missouri farmers consumed 4,385 and 4,989 calories a day, respectively, more than enough calories and protein to perform their arduous work. Researchers compared their daily round of meals with that of urban laborers and decided that "the advantage in diet is in favor of the farm families."[9]

Across the South and up through the Midwest, the anchor of the rural diet was the hog, including all its unctuous by-products. Hog killing took place on the first cold day of autumn, the animals six to eight months old, having spent most of their lives fattening on table scraps and whatever they could find while rooting around the farmyard. In her memoir of Michigan farm life, Della Lutes remembers the grisly splendor of hog-killing day, the sacrificial animal cast in the role of fallen hero. Since everyone kept hogs, the slaughter was repeated day after day, the butchering team moving from farm to farm like a traveling circus. Whole families stood by as the slain animal was suspended, head down, a gambrel stuck through the tendons of its hind legs. A quick slit to the belly and the innards tumbled forth, the "long, undulating convolutions of gray matter" collected in a pan. Each part of the hog was dealt with in turn. The entrails were scrubbed for use as sausage casing; hams, shoulders, and jowls were brined or rubbed with salt and sugar and left to marinate—preparation for their eventual stint in the smokehouse. The "off-fallings" like feet and hocks were simmered clean, the tender scraps of meat returned to the cooking broth and left to jell. The end product was the cold cut known as souse, a reference to the vinegar with which it was seasoned. A similar treatment was extended to the animal's head to make head cheese. The most perishable parts of the animal were consumed by the assembled crowd, the brains scrambled with eggs, the heart and liver fried up and eaten with biscuits and gravy. Even bladders were put to good use—though it wasn't culinary. Rather, they were given to the children, who inflated them, filled them with beans, and used them as rattles. But more valuable than any other by-product was the great reservoir of fat that was "tried out," or rendered. The resulting lard—literally buckets of it—was an everyday staple used for frying, baking, and seasoning. Though each task associated with the slaughter was demanding in its own way, fat rendering offered its own special torments. Despite the unpleasantness, Lutes understood the value of her work:

> *This matter of rendering fat generally lasted over several days and, with its consequent spattering and odor, was one of the least agreeable details of the whole proceeding. Finally, however, when crock after crock was filled with the snowy content, firm and hard, a potential promise of crisp pie crust and smoking friedcakes, as well as exchange matter for groceries, there was that sense of satisfaction in things done that comes to all*

*who by their own hands provide for the physical welfare of
their families.*[10]

No other raw material from the farmhouse cellar received
wider application than those crocks of lard. The cast-iron frying pan liberally seasoned with pork fat never left the stove. The
homemaker reached for it in the morning to fry her eggs and ham,
and again at lunch for the chicken. At supper, she used it to crisp
the cornbread, the batter spooned into a sizzling hot pan, well
greased, before its turn in the oven. In midwestern kitchens, the
lard-based diet achieved its apotheosis in a dish called salt pork
with milk gravy, here served with a typical side of boiled potatoes:

> *On a great platter lay two dozen or more pieces of fried salt
> pork, crisp in their shells of browned flour, and fit for a king.
> On one side of the platter was a heaping dish of steaming pota-
> toes. A knife had been drawn once around each, just to give it
> a chance to expand and show mealy white between the gaping
> circles that covered its bulk. At the other side was a boat of milk
> gravy, which had followed the pork into the frying-pan and
> had come forth fit company for the boiled potatoes.*[11]

Pork fat also found its way into more "delicate" fare. Appalachian
farm women prepared a springtime specialty called "killed lettuce," made from pokeweed, dandelion, and other wild greens
drizzled with hot bacon grease that "killed," or wilted, the tender,
new leaves. The final touch to this fat-slicked salad was a welcome
dose of vinegar.

A farmhouse staple consumed twelve months out of the year
was pie in all its myriad incarnations from rhubarb to mincemeat.
Women baked pies on a daily basis, often three pies a day, one
for each meal, starting with breakfast. With its sugary interior
and lard-enriched crust, a slice of pie in the morning provided

sustained nourishment for a long day's work. At supper, a slice of pie with a cool glass of milk was a fitting reward for a hard day's labor well completed.

These fat-laden dishes, and many more like them, conformed to the rural idea of what food was supposed to be—a concentrated source of energy for men and women who expended it freely. Even in the 1920s, the use of gasoline-powered tractors, balers, and threshers was spreading, but still the exception. In the absence of machines, farmers relied on muscle power, both human and animal. For their wives, the scarcity of electricity and plumbing turned routine housework into daily feats of athleticism, from hauling water, scrubbing laundry, kneading bread, and churning butter to milking the cows and weeding the garden. Conceptions of what constituted a proper meal were grounded in these physical realities, so while the farmhouse menu varied from region to region, the emphasis on sturdy, calorie-heavy food served in large portions remained constant.

No time of year demanded more of those calories than the harvest, the rural busy season. Since the gathering of crops was fueled by human power, neighbor helping neighbor, harvest meals were grand communal events, none more anticipated than the threshing dinners that took place across the Midwest. The wheat harvest was a multistep process that unfolded over a period of days. It began with the cutting of the wheat, which was tied into bundles and left in the fields to dry. On threshing day, the bundles were pitched into wagons and transported to the threshing machine, a great clanky, steam-powered beast operated by a team of traveling threshermen. The job of feeding those men fell to the farmers' wives, teams of women who assembled in each other's kitchens as they followed the threshermen from farmhouse to farmhouse. Culinary preparations began days in advance, with the baking of pies and cakes, half a dozen of each. On the morning of the team's arrival, the women killed and dressed the chickens, baked the bread and biscuits, picked the vegetables, and set them to cook. Beans and beets were boiled, tomatoes stewed, potatoes mashed, and cabbages shredded for coleslaw. The chickens were fried or stewed with dumplings. Cold hams were set onto platters or cut into steaks and fried with drippings. To complete the spread, women descended to their cellars and returned with jams and jellies, home-canned fruit, chow-chows, and pickles. A table was set with places for twenty to twenty-five men, both threshers and neighbors. But before the men could take their seats, the women had them wash at a basin set under a tree beside a stack of clean towels. Since farmhouses had no window screens, the women stood over the eating men, waving leafy branches to shoo away flies. Beneath the swaying branches, the men ate prodigiously, so much so that, to the farmers' dismay, hired hands were immobilized for at least an hour after the meal.

The variety of foods that graced the threshers' table—more than any farmhand realistically needed—expressed in edible form

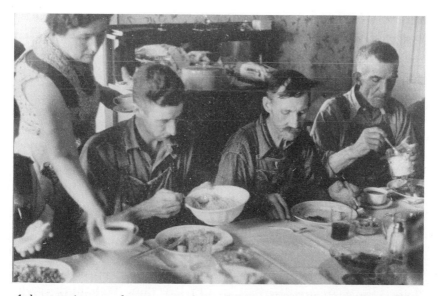

*At harvest time, rural women put their culinary talents on display, preparing meals for teams of threshers, such as these Ohio men.* (Ben Shahn, photographer, Farm Security Administration Collection, Library of Congress, LC-DIG-fsa-8a18590)

the bounty of the season. In winter, however, seasonality had its dark side. The land was not producing, the orchard was bare, and the garden had long since given up its last crop. The bulk of the family's diet was restricted to a regimen of potatoes, meat, beans, and gravy, a diet of necessity, but only up to a point. Women believed that meats, starches, sweets, and fats were the foods that best stoked the human furnace, the culinary antidote to drafty farmhouses in the winter cold. Preserved foods from the cellar helped round out the diet, but the cellar's largess stretched only so far, and by late winter supplies were running alarmingly low. The result was "spring fever," an annual affliction that came on just as the sap began to rise in the trees and that inspired a sprawling body of medical folklore. The ailment, it was thought, resided in the blood, which in spring grew thick with poisons, causing the pulse to slow. Its most telling symptoms were lethargy, muscular weakness, and a bad temper. Women treated it with home-produced "blood tonics" like sassafras tea or sulfured molasses, or they purchased one of the patent medicines concocted exclusively for this particular malady. They understood, however, that the best cure was the first crop of dandelions and spring onions, which were known to thin the blood and revitalize the body. Unknown to them, spring fever was in fact a vitamin deficiency, mostly likely scurvy, brought on by the winter diet.

IN THE LATE 1970s, a group of Indiana farm women, many of them elderly, decided to document their lives as rural homemakers in the first half of the twentieth century. The first volume of their oral history, *Feeding Our Families*, describes the Indiana farmhouse diet from season to season and meal to meal. In the early decades of the century, the Hoosier breakfast was a proper sit-down feast featuring fried eggs and fried "meat," which throughout much of rural American meant bacon, ham, or some other form of pork. In the nineteenth century, large tracts of Indiana had been settled by Germans, who left their mark on the local food culture. A common breakfast item among their descendants was pon haus, a relative of scrapple, made from pork scraps and corn-meal cooked into mush, molded into loaf pans and left to solidify. For breakfast, it was cut and fried. Toward fall, as the pork barrel emptied, the women replaced meat with slices of fried apples or potatoes. The required accompaniment was biscuits dressed with butter, jam, jelly, sorghum syrup, or fruit butter made from apples, peaches, or plums. A final possibility—country biscuits were never served naked—was milk gravy thickened with a flour roux.

To assemble a meal of such complexity meant that women were up and working well before the menfolk, the first chore of the day lighting the woodstove. Beulah Mardis, an Indiana homemaker born around 1900, remembers how her mother timed the morn-ing's biscuits for maximum economy of fuel:

> My mother would build a fire in the stove with wood, she had kindling and she put in about two tablespoonsful of kerosene and two sticks of hickory wood, then she would wash her hands in ice cold water if it was winter, and make the biscuits. By the time the biscuits were mixed, rolled out and cut, and in the pan, the oven was ready and then she would add one more stick of wood in the firebox and that would bake the biscuits. She always said that she baked biscuits on three sticks of wood.[12]

With the oven already hot, the space between breakfast and lunch was time for baking bread, one of many items produced in bulk. For a household of ten, including hired hands, a dozen loaves made every third day was just about adequate. Women pur-chased flour in hundred-pound sacks, two or three at a time, along with ten-pound bags of sugar for use in pies and cakes. However, the one ingredient that never ran out was yeast, a living food that homemakers cultivated in their kitchens and tended like a pet, feeding it regularly with fresh water and starch. The instructions below for "perpetual yeast" come from Adeline Goessling's *Making the Farm Kitchen Pay*:

> *Dissolve one cake compressed yeast in one pint lukewarm unsalted water in which potatoes were boiled. Mix well, add one-half cup sugar, stir thoroughly, pour into a two-quart glass jar, cover loosely and then let stand in a warm place overnight. Next morning it will be a foaming mass. Put the rubber on the can, screw the cover down tight and set away in a cool place. When ready to make bread, pour into the can of yeast foam prepared as above one pint lukewarm water in which potatoes were cooked, mix well, and then stir in one-quarter cup sugar. Let the can stand open in a warm place about five hours, or until the contents are very light and foamy. Then stir it down and use one pint of the mixture for raising four loaves of bread. Put the rubber and cover on the jar again and keep in a cool place. Some of this yeast may be used once or twice a week, or every night, adding fresh potato water and sugar, as described above.*[13]

If the yeast went bad for any reason, women would borrow a cup of healthy yeast from a neighbor and start the process again.

Where farmhouse breakfasts were ample, lunch was more so, especially in summer when workdays were long and appetites pushed to their highest register. With the kitchen garden at full production, the midday meal often included stewed beets, stewed tomatoes, long-simmered green beans, boiled corn, and potatoes fried in salt pork, all cooked to maximum tenderness. At the center of the table often stood a pot of chicken and dumplings, with cushiony slices of white bread to sop up the cooking broth. The gaps between the plates were filled with jars of chow-chow; onion relish; and pickled peaches, cauliflower, and watermelon rinds.

The midday meal concluded with a solid wedge of pie. Like bread, pies were baked in bulk, up to a dozen at a time, and could be consumed at breakfast, lunch, and dinner. The type changed with the seasons, beginning in spring with rhubarb and strawberry and ending in fall with apple. In winter, when the cache of fresh apples was depleted, women made pie from apples they had dried in the fall. Peach and cherry, fruits from the farmer's own orchard, were two summer staples, though women also took advantage of wild blackberries, elderberries, blueberries, and grapes. The following recipe for grape pie comes with no instructions for crust, because every country cook knew how to make that:

Remove the skins from the grapes, bring to a boil and press through a sieve to remove the seeds. Add the skins to the pulp and cook fifteen minutes, then add a cupful of sugar for each two cupfuls of pulp, a tablespoonful of butter and a teaspoonful of corn starch. Bake in a hot oven with two crusts.[14]

When the Indiana homemakers were asked if they ever thought to cut back on all that pie, the women laughed: "A pie was a pie and we ate it and didn't think a thing about it." Did they worry about calories? Certainly not: "We worked, we didn't have to worry about calories."[15] Here was eating at its most transparent, uncomplicated by the food ambivalence that was the plague of "modern," more progressive diners in the Big City.

# Chapter 2

———•·•·•———

OLLOWING THE ARMISTICE, among the Americans returning from Europe was John Dos Passos, a young writer who, like Ernest Hemingway, had served as a volunteer ambulance driver. Dos Passos considered joining the "Lost Generation" of expatriates living in Paris but found the city too "civilized" for him. He returned to New York City, where he sensed that "life, beautiful and cruel, plunges toward new forms of organization."[1] When he landed in New York, Prohibition had just begun and agents armed with billy clubs rifled through his luggage, looking for liquor. Within a few weeks, he was writing to a friend that New York was a combination of ancient Babylon mixed with the harsh aesthetics of the industrial age: "a city of cavedwellers, with a frightful, brutal ugliness about it, full of thunderous voices of metal grinding on metal and of an eternal sound of wheels which turn, turn on heavy stones."[2] Dos Passos later returned to this period in his novel *The Big Money*. In one stream-of-consciousness "Camera Eye" section of the book, his autobiographical narrator remembers his impressions of those early postwar years in New York:

> *and the crunch of whitecorn muffins and coffee with cream gulped in a hurry before traintime and apartment-house mornings stifling with newspapers and the smooth powdery feel of*

*new greenbacks and the whack of a cop's billy cracking a citizen's*
*skull and the faces blurred with newsprint of men in jail.*[3]

The breakfast muffins were a holdover from the era of the Food Administration, which encouraged Americans to "Eat Corn Muffins and Win the War!" because every grain of wheat was being shipped to Europe.

Those first years after the war were also a time of profound unrest and authoritarian reaction. The loosening of wartime wage caps provoked workers from Seattle to Boston to strike for higher pay. Rumors spread that the protests were sparked by Bolshevik agitators hoping to foment a Russian-style revolution, spurring Congress and Attorney General A. Mitchell Palmer to begin a widespread campaign to identify, arrest, and deport any alien "Reds." By 1922, however, any fault lines in American cities had been buried by political repression, the beginning of an unprecedented economic boom, and what Chicago writer Ben Hecht called urban America's "razzle-dazzle of dreams, tragedies, fantasies." Most left-wing agitators were in jail, speakeasies serving illegal booze had replaced saloons, Model Ts crowded the streets, and city dwellers were eager to find new ways to live, work, amuse, and feed themselves.

For both new arrivals and longtime residents, urban life was marked by the challenge of finding a place to live. Apartment leases lasted only a year, usually ending on May 1 or October 1. At the end of that term, the majority of tenants, rich and poor, felt compelled to pack up their possessions and find a new roosting place. On those days, the streets and avenues were clogged with moving vans and even pushcarts piled high with belongings as families headed, they hoped, to newer and cheaper apartments in better neighborhoods. In New York, immigrant families who once crowded the Lower East Side rejected that neighborhood's dingy, claustrophobic, and unhealthy "Old Law" tenements and headed out to new buildings in Brooklyn and the Bronx. Spurred by a servant shortage, middle class families fled their spacious, labor-intensive prewar apartments for a new style of urban living called "efficiency apartments." These were a compromise between hotel and apartment living. In cities such as Boston and New York, residential hotels had long been a popular alternative to rooming houses. They required no leases, so residents could stay for a week, a month, or years; and they also offered the convenience of room service and in-house maids. By the end of the war, however, hotel owners discovered that the new generation of young urbanites wanted the option at least of a modicum of family life. They found a solution by converting their hotel suites into efficiency apartments that offered tenants the cutting edge of technology and maximum convenience.

The hallmarks of the efficiency apartment were "conservation of space, attractive room arrangement and economy of construction."[4] From the central living room, a tenant could reach any part of her apartment in less than ten paces. The compact size allowed builders to maximize the number of units per building and thus their profits. For tenants, it lightened housekeeping chores, eliminating the need for a maid. In order to make the apartments seem more spacious, builders installed the latest in modular, miniaturized, and folding furniture. For sleeping, tenants moved their living room furniture out of the way and pulled Murphy beds out from wall closets. For eating, they could use the Fain Fold-Away Dining Room, a table and two benches that folded out of a wall nook. If they chose to prepare their own meals, they could use the apartment's kitchen, whose compact and highly organized space resembled the meal preparation area in a Pullman dining car.

Kitchenettes, as they were known, came to symbolize the new manners of living and eating in 1920s America. They have their roots in nineteenth-century boardinghouses, where tenants often cooked meals on chafing dishes in their rooms, despite house rules and the obvious fire hazard. Around 1900, urban bohemians began to construct more elaborate pocket cooking areas, dubbed "kitchenettes," for their studios. Seizing on the trend, early household efficiency experts promoted kitchenettes as a way of reducing the drudgery of household tasks, while appliance manufacturers developed a whole new line of products designed specifically for them. By the 1920s, they had become a common element of residential construction projects in vertical cities like New York, St. Louis, and Chicago. At the Surf Apartment Hotel in Chicago, described as "something entirely new in housing accommodations for people of means," the dining area and kitchenette shared a nineteen-by-seven-foot room, with half devoted to the kitchenette. Here's how it was described in a hotel trade journal:

> *The man or woman who designed it was a genius of superlative type for crowding into small space the culinary department of the home. There is a gas range and a gas broiler, these with exhaust vent over. There is a sink five feet long, white enameled. There is a cupboard for ironing board and broom, cupboards for canned foods. There is a major cupboard with many smaller cupboards protected with roll curtain door pulled down over its front. The major cupboard has automatic dust proof bread box, combination flour bin and sifter, automatic sugar dispenser, drawers for knives, forks, and spoons, can openers and the like; a workbench of metal.*[5]

Years before the architect Le Corbusier publicized his phrase, this apartment, and particularly the kitchenette, embodied his belief that "the house is a machine for living."

The young people renting these efficiency apartments lived differently from past generations of city dwellers. They employed no servants, and often both men and women held down full-time

jobs. This, combined with the tiny size of most kitchenettes, necessitated a style of cooking and eating characterized by speed,
economy, and efficiency of space. Homemaking experts who
promoted kitchenettes recognized that a full day of office work
drained women of enthusiasm for the stove. With enough planning and practice, however, they could learn to love kitchenette
cooking: "And if the kitchenette is furnished with attractive-
looking pots and pans and china, and everything is small and
dainty, after the first effort, cooking for herself will soon become
a habit. Next she will be suprized [*sic*] to find how quickly she
becomes a good cook, and what an amount of amusement and
satisfaction will be hers when she asks several friends for dinner,
and cooks the entire meal in the little kitchenette."[6]

Due to poor venting, the first rule was to avoid cooking anything that could generate strong odors, such as onions or cabbage. In the interests of speed and simplicity, manuals like Mabel
Claire's popular *The Busy Woman's Cook Book, or Cooking by the
Clock* (1925) advised women to plan streamlined menus a week
in advance and gave them instructions on how to prepare meals
in thirty, twenty, or even fifteen minutes. These were often built
around three groups of ingredients: dairy products, breads, and
all kinds of canned goods, including soups, vegetables, fruits,
fish, meat, spaghetti, and so on. A typical dinner could be tomato
bisque (soup from a can, with cream added), creamed chipped beef
on toast, a salad of canned string beans with mayonnaise dressing,
and canned fruit topped with whipped cream for dessert. For even
greater efficiency, experts recommended that women equip their
kitchenettes with the newest appliances, including electric perco-
lators, waffle irons, and toasters. Unfortunately, they left unan-
swered the question of where to store them.

In 1921, Irving Berlin memorialized kitchenette living in a
song called "In a Cozy Kitchenette Apartment" for his Music Box
Revue:

*In a cozy kitchenette apartment for two*
*I'll be setting the table*
*While you're cooking a stew for me and you.*
*I'll be there to help you put the dishes away;*
*Then together we'll listen*
*To the phonograph play*
*The tuneful "Humoresque"—*
*And oh, what bliss*
*When it's time to kiss*
*In a cozy kitchenette apartment for two!*[7]

As the decade progressed, however, not everyone who lived in these new apartments found them so blissful. Jane Pride, a writer for the *New York Herald*, described herself as a "kitchenette slave" and declared: "A whole new class of city dwellers, harried, worried, furtive, hungry-looking people, have come into being in the wake of the kitchenette, and no modern influence has had so great a part in affecting the morals, health and spiritual well-being of a generation as has this ill-shapen, ill-planned adjunct of modern living."[8] She realized the room's inadequacy when a deliveryman came with a new appliance and asked, "Where does it go?"

*I pushed aside the blue denim curtain of my kitchenette, reached round and turned on the electric light, and, with a magnificent gesture, indicated about a foot square of floor space and said, "In here—in my kitchen!" The delivery man came and looked. He looked at the ice-box squeezed up against the bag of coals that the Italian "ice, coal and wood man" had just delivered, at the racked shelves, at the two-burner gas stove, huddled on a shelf directly over the ice-box, at the frantic grouping of shelves so that every inch should be occupied by the few pots and pans it was possible to harbor, and then he looked at me. Astonishment fought with pity on his face.*

*"Ain't you got no kitchen?" he asked in the hushed voice of one*
*who might ask: "Ain't you got no parents, little one?"* [9]

Despite the best of efforts of homemaking experts, the reality was that many apartment dwellers did not regularly use their kitchenette's stove. However, they did find uses for its other implements. During Prohibition years, social drinking of bootleg liquor gave far more thrills than serving a good meal; tenants discovered that their kitchenette could serve admirably as a station for mixing drinks:

> *The kitchenette itself is obsolescent in Manhattan. It is as*
> *likely to serve as a cellarette [a kind of mini-bar on wheels],*
> *the presence-chamber, the shrine and the refectory of many*
> *New York suites. Around it at the cocktail hour gathers a de-*
> *voted band which has foresworn its Lares and Penates [Ro-*
> *man household gods] in favor of orange juice, vermouth and*
> *synthetic gin.* [10]

Instead of struggling with the kitchenette, many city residents preferred to purchase ready-made foods for consuming in their dining nook.

With the era of takeout menus and pizza deliverymen still decades in the future, city dwellers who wanted to eat prepared foods bought them at the corner delicatessen, an establishment that has its roots in the nineteenth-century German communities that formed in cities such as New York, Chicago, Milwaukee, and Pittsburgh. In deference to the culinary customs of the Old Country, German delicatessens offered Westphalian hams, North Sea herring (pickled, smoked, and in sour cream), pickles, potato salad, imported chocolates, and so on. The delicatessen business model was soon adopted by German Jewish immigrants, who substituted corned beef and pastrami for the pork products. By the 1920s, delicatessens had broken the boundaries of ethnic neighborhoods and entered the mainstream. In 1921, a Baltimore journalist counted more than fifty delicatessens in his city, calling the imported bologna they sold a "naturalized citizen":

> *It is a natural accompaniment to the new flivver type of kitchen called the "kitchenette," which is just large enough to accommodate a carton of potato salad, a carton of schmierkase, eight inches of wienerwurst, a box of salted crackers and the person designated to prepare the meal, preferably small. Some kitchenettes, larger than others, are built to hold also a pound of boiled ham, sliced thin, and fifteen cents worth of mayonnaise. Others have a larger wienerwurstage. But they all complement the delicatessen store in one way or another.*[11]

Delicatessens lured their customers from the street with a combination of delectable aromas, particularly of pickles and smoked meat, which could reach a pedestrian's nose from half a block away. From a story in the *Saturday Evening Post*, here are the aromas of the fictional Fenstermacher's Delicatessen:

> *Vinegar smell, smell of cheeses, smell of spices, smell of Schmierkase and baked beans on their white enamel trays. Dry smell of packing boxes, caraway seeds and pretzels. Wet smell of near-beer, melting chocolate ice cream, and pickles swimming in flat tubs.*[12]

Inside, delicatessen customers found an eye-popping display of things to eat and drink, all carefully arranged as if by an artist's hand:

*Spices of the Orient render delectable the fruits of the Occident. Peach perches on peach and pineapple, slice on slice, within graceful glass jars. Candies are there and exhibits of the manifold things that can be pickled in one way or another. Chickens, hams and sausages are ready to slice, having already been taken through the preliminaries on the range. There are cheeses, fearful and wonderful, and all the pretty bottles are seen, as enticing looking as ever, although they are but the fraction of their former selves [i.e., under Prohibition].*[13]

Rush hour came in the early evening when commuters, housewives, and children stopped by to pick up something to round out, or make, the evening meal. Sundays were particularly busy, because that was the servants' night off:

*On Sunday night, when we do not need the caution of the commandment that our maidservants shall do no work, then it is that the delicatessen supper comes to its own. Business of transferring the entire contents of the icebox except a few shelves to the dining room table. Business of spreading the festive board until there is no tittle of space except those odd openings that occur when the circumferences of many plates are tangent. Business of mother condescending to heat a few rolls, although that is absolutely all she will have to do with the stove that evening. Business of father sharpening the carving knife raucously and hewing up the ham, let the Saratoga chips fall where they may.*[14]

With the popularity of the delicatessen, however, came the inevitable backlash. Florence Guy Woolston's 1923 story "The Delicatessen Husband" illustrated the perils of the delicatessen lifestyle. Its protagonist, one Perry Winship, grew up in a comfortable, traditional home (complete with his beloved "Ma" in the kitchen) but found a job in the Big City and married Ethel, a career-oriented Vassar graduate. They moved into a "one room, bath, and kitchenette" apartment. Evenings, Perry returns home before Ethel, so it's his job to pick up dinner: "He hated going to the delicatessen. . . . They were emblems of a declining civilization, the source of all our ills, the promoter of equal suffrage, the permitter of business and professional women, the destroyer of the home."[15] What's more, the food is no good, not like Mother used to make. Perry is a victim of circumstances, most of them, it seems, caused by marrying a "modern, self-supporting woman." Ethel cannot cook; hired help either refuse to work in the kitchenette or are so hygienic and "modern" that their food is inedible. So Perry is reduced to standing in line at the delicatessen and juggling the paper-wrapped parcels on the way home, all the time dreaming of the home-cooked meal that might have been: "Cream of asparagus soup, roast stuffed veal, hashed brown potatoes, fresh string beans and old-fashioned strawberry shortcake with whipped cream."

Lingering over this story is the possibility of a 1920s phenomenon called the "delicatessen divorce." Thanks to modern advances, urban apartments needed so little work that the typical "flapper" wife "lolls in bed until nearly noon and then goes down town to shop or to the movies, stops at a delicatessen store and gets something for dinner as she goes home and then thinks she is keeping house."[16] Columnists for the women's magazines told readers that there was no substitute for a home-cooked meal, reminding them that the way to a man's heart was through his stomach.

Despite these proclamations, many city dwellers moved even further away from the kitchen-centered ideal of the American home. "Cafeteria brides" superseded "delicatessen husbands" as many couples and even families simply ate most of their meals out. Instead of struggling to prepare a kitchenette dinner, they enjoyed their evening meals in the nearest cafeteria, which was then a relatively new style of eatery. First appearing in Chicago in the 1890s, cafeterias brought the ideas of modern factory organization and efficiency engineering to the American way of public eating. They dispensed with waiters and replaced them with a self-service system resembling a factory assembly line. Unlike Henry Ford's Model T factories, where the product moved from worker to worker, in cafeterias it was the customers' job to do the moving. They lined up, took a tray, and pushed it along a rail, picking out soup, salad, rolls, entrée, and dessert. Maximizing efficiency, patrons could select food and drink, pay, find a table, and begin eating within a handful of minutes. The further advantages of cafeterias included economical prices, no tipping, and, in the years before Prohibition, a no-alcohol policy, making them suitable for families and young women.

Thanks to cafeterias' low cost and clean image, many nonprofit organizations got into the business, including schools and colleges, YMCAs, Los Angeles vegetarian groups, and the Communist Party, which had a cafeteria on New York City's Union Square. The densest concentration of these restaurants was found in the Los Angeles area, called by wags "Southern Cafeteria." There, big operators like the Boos Brothers built cafeteria empires that offered "quality food, temptingly displayed" in spaces designed more like Hollywood stage sets than simple dining halls. One Boos Brothers cafeteria resembled an old English inn, complete with a half-timbered interior, wrought-iron lanterns, and faux medieval tapestries. The typical meal, however, was all-American. Male customers preferred hearty, meat-centric meals: Swiss steak with gravy, mashed potatoes, cabbage slaw, coffee, and ice cream for dessert. Women, who often made up the majority of the clientele, tended toward lighter dishes such as salads or maybe only a slice of chocolate cake or apple pie à la mode for lunch.

Another inexpensive option for city dwellers was eating in

one of the many "quick lunch" restaurants, also called "gobble-and-git" joints. These eateries often occupied spaces vacated by more traditional restaurants that no longer turned a profit under the dry laws. In New York, the victims included old-time lobster palaces like Rector's and many of the ornate German beer-and-sauerbraten halls. Browne's Chop House, a famous theatrical haunt, was replaced by a Schrafft's. Quick-lunch restaurants substituted the cafeteria steam table with another assembly line of sorts: the lunch counter, which often zigzagged through the interior and was tended by a phalanx of crisp-uniformed waitresses. There the most popular dishes were not hot entrées (though they remained on the menu) but sandwiches and desserts. Before the 1920s, sandwiches were largely confined to picnics and free lunches in saloons and, with their crusts cut off, delicate accompaniments to afternoon tea. With Prohibition and the decade's time-means-money economic boom, office workers turned to sandwiches as the perfect quick and inexpensive lunch.

In 1926, the writer George Jean Nathan counted 5,215 sandwich shops in New York City, 726 in Philadelphia, and 30 in little Altoona, Pennsylvania. Before the 1920s, Nathan claimed that there existed only eight basic sandwich types: Swiss cheese, ham, sardine, liverwurst, egg, corned beef, roast beef, and tongue. In a few short years, however, the creativity of the sandwich makers had reached unprecedented heights: "The sandwich has been brought to a state of variety and virtuosity that has made the standard dishes of the American table seem excessively dull and no longer palatably interesting. There is no taste that the sandwich, in one form or another, cannot gratify." [17] With tongue perhaps slightly in cheek, Nathan claimed that he had counted 946 different sandwich varieties stuffed with fillings such as watermelon and pimento, peanut butter, fried oyster, Bermuda onion and parsley, fruit salad, aspic of foie gras, spaghetti, red snapper roe, salmi of duck, bacon and fried egg, lettuce and tomato, spiced beef, chow-chow, pickled herring, asparagus tips, deep sea scallops, "and so on ad infinitum." Not to be outdone, the Boston writer Joseph Dinneen tallied 1,189 kinds of sandwiches, which he called a natural by-product of modern machine civilization. To meet the demand, bakeries began to make special sandwich-shaped loaves (longer, with flattened tops) for lunch counters, while engineers raced to perfect bread-cutting machines for quicker and more uniform slices. In 1928, the Chillicothe Baking Company of Missouri began selling the first loaves of presliced bread under the Kleen Maid Bread brand. Within a year, bakeries from coast to coast were selling packaged presliced loaves, which were embraced by both lunch counters and housewives as yet another time- and labor-saving convenience.

With their marble tops and lines of rotating stools, lunch counters were installed not only in quick-lunch restaurants but also in drugstores and cigar stores; some were shoehorned into the back of corner candy stores. Here you could get a sandwich or a couple of fried eggs off the griddle, but the real action was centered around the soda fountain, an apparatus that contained soda water spouts, a row of pump dispensers for all kinds of syrups, a freezer where the ice cream was kept, and a row of little tubs filled with chopped fruit, nuts, and other toppings.

The most typical soda fountain concoction was the ice cream soda, which was defined as "a measured quantity of ice cream added to the mixture of syrup and carbonated water."[18] From there, the imaginations of soda jerks were given free range. Trade manuals such as *The Dispenser's Formulary or Soda Water Guide* contained more than three thousand soda fountain recipes for concoctions like the Garden Sass Sundae (made with rhubarb) and the Cherry Suey (topped with chopped fruit, nuts, and cherry syrup). That was just the tip of the fountain iceberg, as soda jerks were constantly inventing new and more eye-popping concoctions. The Oh-Oh-Cindy Sundae, invented by a New London, Connecticut, fountain owner, was made

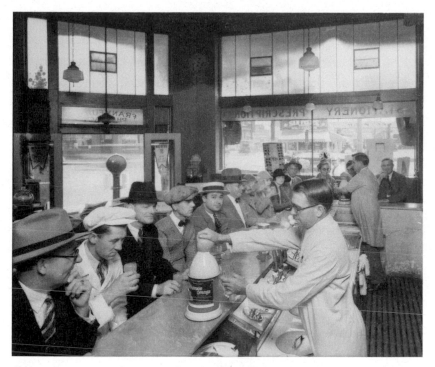

*Convenient counter dining at a Los Angeles soda fountain, 1927.* (Dick Whittington Studio/Corbis)

from strawberry ice cream topped with chocolate syrup, chopped nuts, two ladles of whipped cream, and—for the finish—one red and two green candied cherries. From relatively austere malted milks to the most elaborate sundaes, all of these sweet confections were considered perfectly acceptable as a main course for lunch, particularly by women. In fact, American sugar consumption spiked during the 1920s. This was in part thanks to Prohibition— deprived of alcohol, Americans turned to anything sweet for a quick, satisfying rush—and to the belief that sugar was a relatively healthy "energy" food.

In their kitchen and service operations, the cafeterias, quick-lunch counters, and soda fountains of the 1920s followed the same ideals of industrial efficiency and mass production as Henry

Ford's factories. They differed, however, in the number of products they offered. Ford was famous for making only one auto type, the Model T, which was sold only in black. The typical downtown sandwich counter or soda fountain listed on its menu dozens of products catering to every possible taste. A visit to a Schrafft's, with its menu offering all kinds of soups, hot entrées, salads, sandwiches, ice cream, and cakes, was as much a feature of urban consumer life as walking down Broadway, the buildings ablaze with signs advertising movies, musical shows, toothpaste, burlesque houses, stage shows, nightclubs, coffee, arcades, and so on. And like the Salvation Army preacher on the downtown corner, not everything on the menu was for pure gratification of appetite. A 1928 Schrafft's menu offered "Basy Bread (Reducing)" for fifteen cents an order; Childs restaurant menus listed calorie counts of dishes and added a "V" for vitamins beside any food that was particularly healthy. For breakfast, diners ordered Quaker Oats, containing "protein, carbohydrates, laxative 'bulk' and vitamines, plus toasty creamy deliciousness"; they doused their lunchtime steaks with "Snider's, the vitamin catsup" while drinking Suncrush orange juice containing "all the vitamines and fruit salts so necessary to well-being." Following an aggressive advertising campaign by the Fleischmann's company, they sprinkled yeast into their ice cream sodas to counter "intestinal fermentation," "unsightly skin infections," and "civilization's curse," i.e., constipation. Even sugar was considered a health food, because it would give you the energy to survive the rest of the afternoon in the stenographers' pool.

The 1920s marked the first decade in which science-based concepts of nutrition had an appreciable impact on American food habits. This was particularly true in cities, whose inhabitants had far more exposure to mass media, and mass advertising, than farm families. Up until World War I, most urban and rural Americans based their diet on tradition—if it was good enough for their parents, it was good enough for them—and on what foods were available in local farms and markets. To the extent that people did have an understanding of human metabolism, it was the nineteenth-century idea that the body was a machine, operating something like a steam engine. You simply had to shovel into your stomach enough fuel, or food, to keep the fires burning. The cutting edge of nutrition science was then in Germany, where chemists had developed the tools to analyze and measure the chemical components of meat, vegetables, grains, and other foods. An American scientist named Wilbur O. Atwater imported that technology to the United States and, beginning in 1895, analyzed hundreds of basic American foodstuffs, including corn, beefsteak, turkey, oysters, and apple pie, to discover exactly how much protein, carbohydrate, fat, water, "refuse" (fiber, bones, etc.), "ash" (minerals), and calories they contained. Atwater built an experimental chamber called a respiration calorimeter to study how the human body, at rest and in motion, performing various kinds of work, used those chemicals. He also oversaw a number of studies outside the laboratory to determine the nutrient value of diets consumed by urban workers, university boat crews, African-Americans in Alabama, and other groups. From his research, Atwater developed a worrisome picture of the American diet: Americans spent too much money on food, their dining habits were nutritionally imbalanced, and they generally ate more than they needed. To correct these ills, Atwater held up the traditional New England diet—codfish and potatoes, pork and beans, and bread and milk—as a model to emulate for its emphasis on economy, moderation, and correct nutrition.

The next generation of scientists, however, suspected that Atwater's simple building blocks of fats, carbohydrates, proteins, fiber, and minerals represented only a preliminary understanding of human nutrition. Following Atwater's death in 1907, researchers showed that diseases such as beriberi, scurvy, pellagra, and rickets, once thought to be caused by infectious agents, were likely due to deficient diets. The supposition then was that some elusive "X" factor in food was essential to animal nutrition. One who joined in the hunt for this element was Dr. Elmer V. McCollum, a Kansas farm boy turned biochemist who was among the first researchers to use rats as laboratory test subjects. Around 1912, McCollum devised an experiment to discover if all fats had similar nutritional value (as Atwater surmised) by feeding his rats a diet rich in either butterfat or olive oil. Those that consumed the butterfat grew strong and reproduced, while those that ate the olive oil did not, refuting Atwater's thesis. The nutritional compound extracted from butterfat was dubbed a "vitamine" (a word coined by the Polish chemist Casimir Funk) and specifically "vitamine A," because it was the first of the vitamins to be discovered. It was quickly followed by vitamin B, also known as thiamine (vitamin $B_I$), which is found in whole grains, liver, eggs, and some vegetables.

The link between these scientific discoveries and the foods Americans ate was solidified by the nation's experience during World War I. To feed the troops in Europe, the United States Food Administration under Herbert Hoover began a nationwide propaganda campaign to convince Americans to reduce food waste and eat less wheat, beef, pork, sugar, butter, and other fats. Hoover hired dozens of home economists and nutritionists to promote "Meatless Mondays" and "Wheatless Wednesdays" and come up with alternative foods for American cooks to prepare. These included dishes such as rice flour bread, mutton pie, soybean croquettes, nut and bean loaf with white sauce, and "Wheatless, Eggless, Butterless, Milkless, Sugarless Cake." Government food experts sought to convince consumers not only that eating these concoctions would help win the war but also that they were cheaper, tastier, and more nutritious than the old meat, potatoes, and grain-based staples. Widely distributed government food pamphlets listed the optimal daily calorie counts for men and women at various kinds of work and demonstrated how dried peas, for example, were a perfectly acceptable protein substitute for beefsteak.

The Food Administration also enlisted food scientists such as Dr. McCollum to tour the nation giving talks on the implications of the latest vitamin research for public health, and particularly the raising of children. McCollum's lectures included photos of his laboratory rats. Fed a diet lacking in the "vitalizing element," the first rat was emaciated, with patchy fur and dim eyes. The second, given the scientifically correct blend of nutrients, was long-tailed, glossy-haired, and bright-eyed. Leaping quickly from the world of rats to humans, McCollum told his audience that minuscule doses of certain mysterious chemicals, called vitamins A and B, were necessary for a healthy life. Without them, adults would become susceptible to many diseases and, worse, the young would "suffer, grow weak and sickly." Luckily, McCollum had discovered the solution, which was to replace the old meat, potatoes, bread, and sugar diet with one that was rich in leafy greens and, most important, dairy. For McCollum, consuming milk, butter, and cheese was not only nutritionally wise but a patriotic duty: "Who are the peoples who have achieved, who have become large, strong, vigorous people, who have reduced their infant mortality, who have the best trades in the world, who have an appreciation for art and literature and music, who are progressive in science and every activity of the human intellect? They are the people who have patronized the dairy industry." [19]

Following the end of World War I, the Food Administration was quickly disbanded, while Herbert Hoover hustled off to Europe to oversee food relief. Some food scientists, nutritionists, and home economists moved over to the USDA's Bureau of Home Economics, where they concentrated their work on studies of vitamins, food composition, and diets of various groups. Others returned to their home states to find work in education, magazines, newspapers, restaurants, and food manufacturing. In their new positions, they continued to promote the gospel that the key to good health was eating the correct food. The basis of their argument was the latest scientific research on vitamins, calories, minerals, and the workings of the human digestive system. However, this message was often filtered through other aspects of their work. In science, vegetarians found proof that eating meat was not only unnecessary for human health but also unnatural. The Borden company used science as a selling point for its condensed milk (made with "country milk and pure sugar"), which was recommended by doctors for babies who were "undernourished, weak and underweight." The *New York Herald Tribune* published articles promoting Branzos, a Purina bran product, which contained, according to scientific analysis, "valuable minerals (for teeth and bone building) and phosphorus (for the growing and active cells of the vital organs, such as liver, brain, and nervous tissues)."[20] The result was a multiplicity of voices—from the family doctor to the goateed specialist in the Fleischmann's yeast ad, the newspaper cooking editor, and the pamphleteer on the street corner—all claiming to have authoritative answers to the pressing question "What to eat?"

For those most closely tied to the nutritional "establishment"— food scientists and home economists affiliated with large research institutions—the solution was the "balanced diet," achievable only by consuming the correct quantities of proteins, carbohydrates, fats, minerals, and vitamins. Some of this information came from the Bureau of Home Economics, which after the war published a few pamphlets on food choice and child nutrition. Much more of it was generated by college home economics departments and distributed through home economics classes in both rural and urban schools, books, newspapers, and magazine articles. For example, in 1926, *Good Housekeeping* published an article called "Guide Posts to Balanced Meals" that synthesized the scientific consensus on the balanced diet down to six easily digested points:

*Balance your meals for the day as follows:*

1. *One pint of milk a day as either a beverage or partly in soups, sauces or desserts.*
2. *Two generous servings of non-starchy vegetables (such as carrots, lettuce, spinach, string beans, cabbage, beets), at least one of these raw whenever possible.*
3. *One serving of fresh fruit, raw if possible.*
4. *One moderate serving of meat, or a meat substitute such as a cheese or egg dish.*
5. *One egg a day in addition to this.*
6. *To make up the energy requirement for the day add breads (including whole wheat), starchy vegetables (such as potatoes and baked beans), cereals (including whole grains), desserts, butter and cream.*[21]

As a simple yet scientifically based guide to eating for health, this was an ancestor to the federal government's more recent charts featuring various food pyramids and plates.

During the 1920s, however, the balanced diet was far from the last word on human nutrition. From radio to newspapers to advertising, the media were filled with self-declared diet experts claiming to have the best answer to the question of what to eat. One strain of this discourse was devoted to the perils of certain food combinations. Balanced diet proponents recommended eating a wide variety of foods; food combination alarmists claimed this would surely cause injury. According to Dr. William Porter of New York, "Ninety per cent of all human ailments, apart from disorders incident to old age and acute infections, are due to wrong combination and foolish food selection."[22] One proponent of this theory announced that meat and bread should never be eaten together, because "their modes of digestion are so different that they are quite incompatible."[23] Another believed that milk, meat, and bread together made the perfect combination. All seem to have agreed that fruits and "acid" vegetables should be kept as far away from starchy foods as possible. If one made the mistake of eating, say, spaghetti with tomato sauce, the combination would cause fermentation in the digestive tract and, inevitably, souring of the blood, aka acidosis. Acidosis, a high acid level in the blood, is today usually diagnosed as due to overexercise or pulmonary problems. In the 1920s, acidosis was named the culprit for everything from general lack of pep to bouts of vomiting in children. To prevent this scourge, a group called the Defensive Diet League of America handed out a chart showing lists of acid- and alkali-forming foods and advising that the ideal diet should be made of 20 percent acid foods and 80 percent alkali foods. Some doctors protested that many cases ascribed to acidosis were probably due to food poisoning, but their voices were lost in the din.

Indeed, the 1920s were probably the high point of food faddism in the United States. Dietary evangelists of one stripe or another touted the health benefits of fasting, mastication, vegetarianism, fruitarianism, raw foods, sour milk, drinking two quarts of milk daily, the grape cure, no breakfast, no protein, hot water, no water with meals, coffee with meals, liver as a miracle food, and on and on. Many of these programs were supposed to enhance not only internal well-being but external beauty as well. After centuries of judging the curvaceous form ideal, millions of American women suddenly decided that the slim, "sylphlike," and boyish body type was now the goal. They embarked on all kinds of reducing regimens, including the canned pineapple and lamb chop diet, supposedly popular among movie stars: "For breakfast the order is one lamb chop and one slice of pineapple. For luncheon two lamb chops and one slice of pineapple. For dinner two lamb chops and two slices of pineapple."[24] That combination of meat and fruit was somehow supposed to melt the pounds away. In fact, so many women—and more than a few men—were experimenting with drastic diets, high colonics, patent medicines, therapeutic soaps, and other nostrums guaranteed to shed pounds that thousands were ending up in hospitals, victims of physical and mental collapse. Alarmed, in 1926 the American Medical Association convened an "Adult Weight Loss Conference" in New York with leading doctors as speakers. After the conference, they drafted a widely reprinted, sixteen-part series of articles exposing the dangers of reducing fads and recommending a gradual plan consisting of exercise and a balanced, low-calorie diet. Their efforts mainly fell on deaf ears. At the end of the decade arose the Hollywood Diet, featuring a menu of grapefruit and various proteins and guaranteed to help you lose eighteen pounds in as many days. Once again, hospitals saw a rise in "cases of acidosis, jaundice, anaemia and similar complaints arising from malnutrition from its adherents" and issued a new series of health warnings.

Despite the prevalence of trendy diets and new systems of eating, there was a limit to what urban diners would tolerate. One restaurateur who discovered this was William Childs, one of the founders of the Childs restaurants. In 1889, he and his brother opened their first restaurant in New York City, offering quick service, low prices, spotless sanitation, and simple but filling dishes. By the 1920s, the company had grown to a chain of more than 120 restaurants nationwide serving 52 million meals a year, mainly to office workers, efficiency apartment dwellers, and downtown shoppers. William Childs was a health nut, however, and also a vegetarian who believed that the nation's meat-eating days were numbered. Starting in 1920, he began to remove meat dishes from his menus (corned beef hash was the last to go), replacing them with concoctions like meatless meat loaf and beefless beef stew. He added vitamin and calorie counts to the menu, along with profiles of famous vegetarians in history. Unfortunately, the dining public did not share his enthusiasm and began to transfer their patronage to other restaurants. When Childs shares began to plummet, stockholders rebelled, demanding that "Mr. Childs cut out his other fads and feed the feeder what he wants."[25] Childs was forced to resign, and the vegetarian menu was discarded and replaced by one heavy in beef stew, veal cutlets, roast pork, and bacon. With meat back on the menu, customers returned to Childs.

During the 1920s, changes to the urban diet were so rapid and capricious that many food businesses feared they could not keep up. Nineteenth-century food habits had been left behind, but it was hard to discern where American diners were heading. To help manufacturers chart a course, in 1929, Christine Frederick published a book called *Selling Mrs. Consumer*, aimed squarely at companies that sold food, appliances, cosmetics, clothes, and furniture to American women. Frederick, a popular home economics writer and lecturer, dedicated her book to Herbert Hoover, the newly elected president, who had acted as secretary of commerce under Presidents Harding and Coolidge. At Commerce, Hoover had revitalized a moribund department and helped rationalize American business, build new markets, and find hundreds of new ways to measure economic activity. Inspired by his work, Frederick believed that women consumers were a key but often ignored segment of the American economy. Her book aimed to convince businesses of the importance of the women's market and to tell them exactly what kind of dresses, toasters, and foodstuffs women would be likely to buy.

Digging deeply into reams of government statistics, Frederick

attempted to elucidate American dining habits past, present, and
future. Her work focused on urban consumers, because she believed it was only a matter of time before rural Americans would
eat, dress, and furnish their homes the same as city dwellers. At
the time, 27 percent of the average household budget was spent on
food (versus 13 percent today). Frederick noted that consumption
of meat, potatoes, and bread—the staples of nineteenth-century
America—was dropping, as were sales of "poverty staples" such as
salt pork, salt beef, molasses, and cornmeal. In place of old, heavy,
time-consuming, multicourse meals, Americans were now eating
fewer courses of lighter foods that were actually more expensive
because they had often been imported from other regions or even
overseas. Meals included markedly more fruits and green vegetables (both fresh and canned), more milk and dairy products,
and much more sugar, candy, soda, and ice cream. The reasons for
these changes included more sedentary lives, fewer servants, more
women in the workforce, and a greater emphasis on nutrition and
dieting. Unlike their rural counterparts, urban women no longer
defined themselves by the quality of their cooking:

> At one time eating was Mrs. Consumer's "indoor sport" or
> amusement, or at least a pastime in those dark eras before the
> auto, the movie, the radio, and other inventions came to pro-
> vide more interests. Undoubtedly for this reason women no lon-
> ger cook so abundantly and so often. For them, too, cooking used
> to be a social accomplishment, one of the few creative expres-
> sions in that drab era when girls remained girls and daugh-
> ters faced a life choice between marrying or entering a convent.
> What else was there for a woman to do?[26]

In the decade to come, Frederick divined that these trends would
only continue, with even greater consumption of fruit, vegetables,

dairy products, and imported foods. Custom and habit would no longer dictate what dishes were served; women would select food for "style," which Frederick defined as "related to flavor, novelty, appearance, and unusual modes of service." The days of the country store, with its big barrels of flour, sugar, and other raw ingredients, were numbered; women would demand foods that were processed and packaged "to save time, effort or fuel in their preparation."[27] Interest in the "health, vitamin and beauty appeals" of various foodstuffs would not only continue but become the defining factor in food preparation. In her lectures, Frederick defined the difference between the past and future of American dining as the difference between "cooking" and "feeding." For her, cooking was one of the primitive arts, going back to the caveman dragging a dead buck back to the cave for his wife to prepare: "And she, bending low, with constant basting and turning and watching of the fire, gave it undivided attention for hours. This is *cooking*."[28] In contrast, the housewife of the future would concentrate on feeding, much like the farm girl feeding her prize pig its rations:

> *This girl gave her "Buster" just precisely so much cornmeal to eat, just so much buttermilk, just so much shorts; carefully measured amounts and kinds of foods at proper intervals,— foods that were selected for definite nutritive value. Her prize pig received "rations," or a "balanced meal," and became a prize pig because he was fed, and not merely cooked for! "Feeding," and not "cooking" has long been the slogan of the stock raiser desirous of producing a prize pig or any other animal. But it is only very recently that the housewife has learned to feed her family, and stop just cooking for it. Feeding implies a knowledge of nutritive values, while cooking implies nothing more than an appeal to taste.*[29]

The days of "cooking" such as practiced by rural homemakers were numbered. In the future, American families would be "fed" with nutritive products guaranteed to make children healthier and more vigorous, and housewives slimmer and more beautiful. Any connection to glossy and bright-eyed laboratory rats or pigs being fattened up for the slaughter was presumably coincidental.

# Chapter 3

———◦———

AMONG THE BEVY of attractions that New York offered early twentieth-century tourists was the spectacle of the city's breadlines. Helpfully listed in period guidebooks, the breadlines operated between midnight and 1 a.m., when legitimate forms of entertainment had wrapped up for the evening. Viewers who came to the breadlines expecting delinquent behavior left dissatisfied. Patrons of the line seemed to materialize all at once, and from all directions, providing opportunity for at least some minor shoving, yet confrontations were rare. Well bundled against the cold, onlookers took careful note of the men's sinking posture, their frayed and insubstantial clothing, and their overall demeanor, catching stray fragments of conversation whenever possible to see what these individuals had to talk about. The action reached its climax when a light flickered on inside the kitchen, the men bolted to attention, and the line surged forward. Thirty minutes later the crowd had dissipated, some with bread stuffed in their pockets, and the street was empty.

What the breadline lacked in more conventional sightseeing appeal, it made up for in sociological interest, part of a larger Progressive Era commitment to open the shutters on urban poverty. Jacob Riis gave this impulse a rallying cry with the title of his 1893 book, *How the Other Half Lives,* an illustrated foray into the New York slums in all their manifold wretchedness. On the misery index, however, no population was considered worse off than the men on the breadline, which, for inquiring tourists, only added to its allure. The terrific humiliation of begging for food was an option for only the most unfortunate or, conversely, the most degenerate characters, and people argued for both. The clash of perspectives was one facet of a much larger conversation about the poor and how they should be treated. Among the upper classes, it was generally assumed that the poor fell into one of two camps, those deserving or undeserving of charity, a distinction that went all the way back to the English poor laws. Among the deserving were widows and orphans, the aged, feebleminded, and infirm—in other words, victims of bad luck. The undeserving, by contrast, were morally corrupt, naturally inclined to boozing, gambling, and loafing. Disagreement over where to place the "breadliners" was a point of debate among both casual spectators and professional social workers, people trained to make that diagnosis. How they were classified determined how they should be treated, whether they should be fed or sentenced to forced labor. (The novelist Theodore Dreiser was a proponent of labor camps, his conclusion after spending time on the breadline during his research for *Sister Carrie*.)

The city's first long-standing breadline was attached to the ultrafashionable Vienna Model Bakery, a café on East Tenth Street owned by Louis Fleischmann of the Fleischmann's yeast dynasty. Founded on the idea that the hungry deserve to eat, no questions asked, Fleischmann's breadline carried on for a good two decades, serving as the model for a string of imitators. Administered by evangelical groups like the Salvation Army, the new breadlines were sensibly clustered along the Bowery, close to the men they intended to serve. Already a nesting ground for the unemployed, the Bowery at the start of the twentieth century was home to a distinctive urban ecosystem. Relics of the old Bowery, the city's main entertainment street going all the way back to the

Civil War, survived in the scattering of theaters, honky-tonks, and dime museums that now catered mainly to tourists. (After a midnight visit to the breadline, out-of-towners could repair to one of the Bowery beer saloons, often with a hired police escort, to round out the evening.) The Bowery's main business, however, was homelessness. Bowery habitués were typically drifters. Unencumbered by wives or children, May through November they scoured the countryside tracking down work as bridge builders, canal diggers, loggers, and farmhands, migrating to the Bowery when cold weather hit and jobs dried up. Here, under the shadow of the elevated railroad, they relied on a network of cheap lodging houses, saloons, employment agencies, and five-cent lunch counters to survive the winter. For a free shave, they paid a visit to one of the Bowery barber colleges. To raise cash, they hocked whatever possessions they could live without at one of the local pawnshops.

When their cash ran out, which it inevitably did, the men traded in their ten-cent beds for improvised shelter in alleyways, in stairwells, and on park benches under tented blankets of newspaper. For food, they turned to the breadlines, receiving midnight portions of dry bread and coffee, which the charities euphemistically referred to as a "promenade breakfast." The reason they served it at such an ungodly hour, charity officials explained, was to ensure that all takers were legitimately destitute, as no one with a bed to sleep in would rouse himself for such meager rewards. While Bowery Missions said all men were worthy, the midnight breakfasts suggested that worthiness was relative, the meal providing sustenance and punishment in near equal proportions.

The Bowery breadlines, up and running between Thanksgiving and Easter to accommodate the winter influx, were catnip for newspapermen. Borrowing from the moviemaker's tool kit, reporters used panning shots, close-ups, and the occasional montage to create stories that unfolded like cinematic shorts. A 1908 article on the Bowery Mission from the *New York Times* contains the following set piece:

> *Down through the open door came the army of the poor to the coffee and the rolls, tramping, tramping. The pallid faces of them! The hands outstretched for the rolls, the trembling lips pressed to the heat of the coffee in the cups. The misshapen hands, the grimy hands, the long, attenuated fingers, the cold, blue lips, the wolfish, backward look of the wild eyes at the pile of rolls, the fiendish stare of insatiable and unsatisfied hunger.*[1]

Here were the breadliners at their most menacing, but even more sympathetic portrayals left a similar impression of otherness. Whether born that way or beaten down by circumstance, or some combination of both, the men on the line followed their own code of behavior, spoke in their own dialect, and generally kept to themselves, observing the invisible boundary that isolated the Bowery from the city around it.

When the economy stumbled, which it did in the panic of 1907, the breadlines grew to maximum length (that year the Bowery Mission fed more than 2,500 men a night) and made headline news until the markets recovered and lines shrank to their normal size. Public interest spiked a second time in 1918 when the sudden drop in production after the war combined with the flood of returning soldiers to cause high unemployment. Both downturns were just two in the long chain of depressions and recessions, periods of inflation and deflation, that the United States had weathered over the decades.

In the 1920s, beginning under Calvin Coolidge, the country experienced a six-year stretch of breakneck economic expansion. Factories were running full tilt and at increased efficiency, churning out a parade of new goods. With the encouragement of an emerging advertising industry, Americans clamored for the latest contraptions, spending freely on everything from electric vacuum cleaners to automobiles. What they couldn't afford outright, they purchased on the installment plan, another of the period's innovations. While consumers swooned, American businesses aspired to a new a scale of operation, the nation's larger concerns swallowing up their junior counterparts to form some of the country's first publicly owned corporations. All appearances suggested that the cycle of boom and bust had run its course.

Intoxicated by the new prosperity, Herbert Hoover, who was running for president in 1928, famously announced that America was "nearer to the final triumph over poverty than ever before in the history of any land." Unfortunately, Hoover's calculation rested on an oversight: The distribution of America's new wealth was severely lopsided, the overwhelming share flowing directly into the bank accounts of the very rich, leaving the poor with few or no gains at all. Among the excluded were the seasonal workers who wintered on the Bowery. However, by this time the general public had become acclimated to the vagrants, accepting them as permanent figures. Commotion over the breadlines had also died down. Operating under cover of night, in neighborhoods that most New Yorkers avoided, they were easily ignorable, a luxury that ran out with the end of the decade.

Through the spring and summer of 1929, confidence in the limitlessness of America's newfound wealth had taken hold of Wall Street, driving stocks into the stratosphere. Suspended there by sheer faith, stock values needed only a loss of confidence to go plummeting back to earth. The stock market crash, conventionally pinned to October 29, was not in fact a single event but a series of falls and recoveries that unfolded over a period of weeks. Prices on Wall Street began to coast downward in early September and continued their measured descent until October 19, when volume surged and prices tumbled. Over the next two days, Wall

Street seemed to steady itself, but on October 23, the semblance of order evaporated, and in the final hour of trading stock prices plummeted. Primed by the end-of-the-day slide, speculators were ready to sell from the minute the market opened the following day. When no buyers materialized, stocks went into free fall. The apprehension of the previous few days now crossed over into outright panic. Like a slow-motion demolition, the collapse resumed on October 29 and shuddered to something like a conclusion a week later, on November 4.

After the crash, a "fog of war" effect settled over the United States, obscuring conditions on the ground so that even the most basic economic facts were in dispute. Statistics acquired a new slipperiness. Government estimates on unemployment jumped from one extreme to the other, depending on who was bearing the news. After several nervous months, in January President Hoover announced that the employment tide had turned. All the major industries were gathering speed and the jobless were finding work. Certain that the president's numbers were off, Frances Perkins, who was then industrial commissioner of New York, responded with her own analysis. According to her presumably more accurate figures, employment in New York, a bellwether for the rest of the country, was at its lowest levels since 1914, the year that record keeping began. Further confounding the picture, a third set of numbers, collected by the New York Board of Trade, indicated that the local employment crisis had crested and that a spring bounce back was imminent.

But in New York City, in place of the warm-weather turnaround, the breadlines made an unscheduled appearance. Jobless workers took up their posts at all the old Bowery charities: only this was exactly the time of year when breadlines were supposed to be shutting down for the season. So this was odd. It appeared—although no one was too sure—that New York's vagrant population, discouraged by gloomy work prospects out in the countryside, had decided to stay put and spend the summer in town. More unsettling, however, was that *new* breadlines were popping up, and in the best neighborhoods, a piece of tramp culture broken free of its natural habitat, now at large in the wider city.

The sight of those renegade lines tore through the politicians' chatter like a shard of glass through a silk veil. In March, in the city's most elegant retail district, Fifth Avenue shoppers were startled by a trail of hungry men leading to the Church of the Transfiguration (also known as the Little Church Around the Corner) on East Twenty-Ninth Street. Like an apparition, the line seemed to grow before their eyes, the number of men doubling every few days until it was a solid wall of humanity, five abreast, which wrapped clear around the block. Local merchants, worried about the breadline's effect on shopper morale, were predictably distraught. When they complained to the city, Mayor Jimmy Walker threatened to

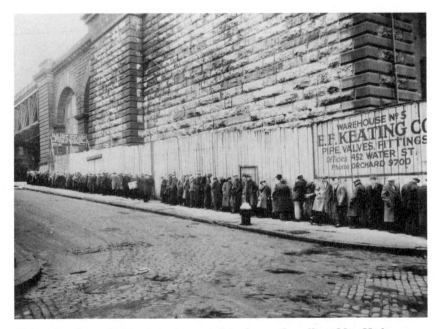

*Unemployed men biding their time on a Manhattan breadline, New York, 1930.*
(Library of Congress, LC-USW33-035391-ZC)

arrest the church rector, Dr. Randolph Ray, for creating a public disturbance.

Whereas religious institutions were old hands in the bread-line business, that spring diverse New Yorkers started their own breadlines, soup kitchens, and food distribution depots. Political clubs, business associations and fraternal orders, debutantes and socialites, newspaper publishers, veterans' and religious groups, and even the occasional crime boss all mobilized, establishing makeshift charities for feeding the hungry. By the start of 1931, the city had eighty-two standing breadlines, the number mis-leadingly low, as lines opened and folded every few weeks or even days, bringing the total number deep into the hundreds. Collectively, the lines served roughly 85,000 meals a day, which begged the question: If business was "on a sound footing," as Hoover maintained, and Americans were fruitfully employed, who were all these hungry people?

Following their turn-of-the-century predecessors, reporters engaged in a kind of breadline semiotics, reading the men's outer shells for signs of their identity. At a time when a man's wardrobe encoded his biography, the sartorial diversity found on the lines was newsworthy in its own right:

> *Men with overcoats, men without, men with dirty sweaters buttoned close around dirtier necks; men with nothing warmer than a summer suit of cheap cotton stuff; men with the collars of two flannel shirts sticking out; men with nothing but a cotton shirt and a jumper blouse to keep out the cold of yesterday. Old men, the usual type of Bowery Bum; "dopes," "rummies," "lush divers," who sidle along with furtive glances. . . . Young men with Scandinavian blondness who weave along as though they still walked the decks of the ships where they can't find seamen jobs because the town is flooded with their kind. In that hungry line one finds by questioning a few walks of every type*

*of worker. There are laborers, carpenters, roofers, bakers, fore-*
*men, engineers, toolmakers, railroad workers, waiters, cooks,*
*pantrymen, cigar makers, metal polishers, bricklayers, pipefit-*
*ters, garage men, chauffeurs. There are common laborers, men*
*with trades and men of the white collar class . . . shaved and*
*equipped with clean linen.*[2]

Those white collars became the story within the story. To observers, they stood out from the crowd like doves among pigeons, the
people inside them objects of special sympathy—an irony, as this
was precisely what the men were trying to fend off.

To prop themselves up, former office workers, humiliated by
their sudden reversal, dressed for the breadline in full white-collar
regalia—a clean shirt, a respectable suit, and, of course, a proper
hat—a "bold haberdashery front" their best insulation against the
indignity of joining the line. On a more practical note, the right
clothes increased a man's chances of landing a job for the future.
Since the jobless spent hours a day shuttling from one employment agency to the next, it was imperative to dress the part of
the bookkeeper, engineer, or ad man. With so much riding on
appearances, men (or more precisely their wives) treated work
clothes like family heirlooms. Shirts were laundered, suits were
pressed and kept in working order—no buttons missing—hence
the unlikely spectacle of breadliners dressed as though on their
way to a business lunch.

Under no central command, each of the city's breadlines devised its own strategy for feeding the multitudes. Those of limited means put out the call for donations, of both cash and in
kind. In Greenwich Village, the Sisters of Charity at St. Vin-
cent's Hospital served three meals a day with food donated by
neighborhood businesses, including bread and crullers from the
local Horn & Hardart. Further uptown, in his Sunday sermon,

Pastor Adam Clayton Powell pledged four months' salary to a basement soup kitchen for his Abyssinian Baptist Church. His topic that morning, the appetite of a hungry God. In these hard times, he preached, the way to appease a hungry God was to do like his only son and tend to the needs of the body, filling men's stomachs as well as their souls. The congregation responded by storming the pulpit with pledges and donations of their own. Between Christmas and Easter of that year, the church served 28,500 free meals, sending out 2,125 basket dinners and distributing 1,530 pieces of bread and pastry, each portion duly recorded by the church secretary.

Meanwhile, at the high end of the income spectrum, some of New York's wealthiest citizens funded breadlines by reaching into their personal bank accounts. Marian Spore was a Park Avenue socialite with an unusual hobby as a "psychic" artist. Untrained by conventional means, she received tutoring of an original sort, painting under the guidance of spirits. Spore was also active in charity, though not in the check-writing way typical of her Park Avenue crowd. Instead, twice a week, she was chauffeured to the Bowery, where she set up shop on a quiet corner, handing out free meal tickets redeemable at the YMCA cafeteria just a few blocks away. Spore's technique for dispensing charity, similar to her painting, made use of her intuitive faculties. One penetrating glance at the figure before her was all she required to determine the extent of his needs, no questions necessary. The average customer received a total of four tickets, each worth a nickel, while those she perceived as real hard-luck cases walked away with "a long strip of uncounted tickets in their shaking hands." The city's flashiest food charity was sponsored by publishing magnate William Randolph Hearst, who enlisted two army trucks, loaded them with edible hand-outs, and parked them in the two most conspicuous locations he could find—namely Times Square and Columbus Circle. Day and night (after dark they were lit with klieg lights), the Hearst trucks attracted a zigzagging line of New Yorkers, often waiting for hours, for free sandwiches, doughnuts, crullers, and coffee.

Finally, to maximize their reach, the breadlines entered into partnerships with a select group of New York restaurants, cheap lunchrooms patronized almost exclusively by men, where customers could fill up—and do it quickly—on a twenty-cent tab. So, at the Little Church Around the Corner, roughly a thousand men a day received meal tickets to Beefsteak John's, an old-time eating house with several outposts on the Bowery. The Salvation Army devised a similar system, handing out tickets to the kind of no-frills restaurants favored by the traditional Bowery crowd.

With only a single exception, the proliferation of breadlines during that first winter of the Great Depression was an improvised response by private charities and individuals to a growing food emergency. The one outlier was the line sponsored by the Municipal Lodging House, an institution dating back to the nineteenth century that provided homeless New Yorkers with a bed and two meals a day. The 1886 law that brought the lodging house into existence stipulated that the content of those meals be "plain and wholesome," the two hardest-working adjectives in American culinary history. *Plain* was no understatement. For its first twenty-five years, the Municipal Lodging House fed guests on a regimen of oatmeal, bread, tea, and coffee. After 1900, as the emerging science of nutrition progressed, public charities responsible for feeding both the poor and the sick were increasingly indebted to "food standards," scientifically determined recommendations for the quantity of food required by the body.

In 1917, the New York City Department of Welfare issued its own food standards, or "Basic Quantity Food Tables," a separate table for each population under its care. Drawing heavily on Wilbur O. Atwater's nutritional research, the standards took into account such objective variables as age, sex, occupation, and, importantly, food cost. More intangible factors, however, slipped into the calculus. Doctors who worked at city hospitals, for example, were better fed than nurses, who were better fed than orderlies. The 1917 food standards enlarged the lodging house menu so it now included a bowl of soup for supper. But even with that addition, in the city's nutritional hierarchy municipal lodgers were a step under prison inmates, the least deserving of basic nourishment.

The expanded menu did little to entice the homeless, who bristled at the various demands imposed by the "Muni," starting with the interrogation administered to all guests upon their arrival. They resented the half day of obligatory labor—either cleaning the building or chopping wood—that was known as a "work test," an attempt to determine if the men were worthy of charity. What they dreaded most, though, were the mandatory baths, an insult to the hoboes' sense of independence and, as far as they were concerned, a waste of time and energy. A 1923 headline from the *New-York Tribune* neatly summed up the men's position: "Tired Hobo's Last Resort Is City's Lodging House, for There He Has to Bathe." Rejected by its intended clientele, the lodging house was chronically short on guests, a state of affairs that persisted through the 1920s. By the spring of 1930, however, with unemployment climbing and jobless out-of-towners streaming into the city, the eight hundred lodging house beds were inadequate to serve the growing number of homeless. The city responded by opening two annexes, each one with double the capacity of the original.

All three shelters were under the command of an especially dedicated and talented public servant, a World War I veteran named Joseph Mannix, who moved himself, his wife, and three young daughters into the main building on East Twenty-Fifth Street. From there, Mannix directed a kind of clearinghouse for the homeless, providing them with a clean bed for the night along with a broad range of social services. For nourishment, guests received two meals a day, breakfast and supper. At lunchtime, Mannix presided over the city's most patronized breadline. The municipal dining room, open to anyone willing to endure the wait, was housed in a converted warehouse on a pier on the East River. The line for the "mayor's dining room" began to form at nine in the morning. At eleven, it was open for business. The municipal menu rotated between beef and mutton stew, franks and beans, and, on Fridays, clam chowder, all entrées served with a half pound of sliced bread. Cooked in sixty-gallon vats, the food was served cafeteria-style in pressed aluminum dishware and carried on aluminum trays to the double row of picnic tables that ran down the center of the long dining hall. As each man rose from his spot on the bench, a new one took his place.

However they managed to operate, breadlines throughout the city adhered to a common culinary vision. The pillars of the breadline kitchen were beef, bread, coffee, and sugar, a throwback diet that ignored the many pronouncements about calories, vitamins, and food groups that had dominated nutritional thinking in the 1920s. Providing well-balanced meals, however, was not in the sights of breadline organizers. Instead, breadlines offered emergency rations, foods that were cheap, filling, familiar, and satisfying, and never meant for long-term consumption. From the start, breadlines were a stopgap measure intended to tide people over until prosperity was restored.

Photographs of the breadlines captured the plight of the jobless in a single image. The rivers of hunched men in dark overcoats and battered hats, endlessly reproduced in newspapers and magazines, suggested that hunger was confined to unemployed men, and that women, who were back at home with the kids, were managing on their own. In reality, women across urban America—in fact, a quarter of the American workforce—now earned their living outside the home. Included in those numbers were the many thousands of country girls who had left the family farm to find jobs as waitresses, store clerks, factory hands, and office workers. However they were employed, as the economy unraveled, women, too, lost their jobs, and at a quicker rate than men. The fact that women were missing from the breadlines was never a reflection of need. Rather, women were barred from the lines by force of social convention. In a sad irony, no one observed this particular convention more faithfully than the people it harmed most directly. "Business girls"—young, unattached women employed as typists, switchboard operators, bookkeepers, and stenographers—now suddenly jobless, resisted the breadlines no matter how dire their situation.

To a woman of the 1930s, the breadlines, like any other charity, carried the stigma of poverty, only here the humiliation was multiplied by the very public nature of the lines. This particular charity, moreover, was created for men, and an especially rough class of men at that. Women had no place in an all-male dining hall, sharing tables with strangers, many with coarse manners and disreputable histories. For a woman, to be caught in the breadline milieu was to place her good character in question. To accommodate the women's sense of propriety, a handful of all-female breadlines were established, but they never gained traction. One of them, a midtown storefront that called itself the Good Samaritan, served free coffee and sandwiches in a "dainty" dining room complete with "women's sized tables." But despite the ladylike decor and the deliberate use of window curtains for shielding the women from passersby, would-be customers paced the sidewalk outside the establishment, holding their meal tickets, reluctant to cross the threshold.

The single woman who accepted charity confirmed—both to herself and to everyone around her—that she was truly alone in the world with no man to support her, a stigma that remained in force despite women's new freedoms. As one social worker explained it, "There is something about standing in a breadline that makes it seem almost impossible. . . . Women still carry in their minds psychological remnants of the Age of Protection; to admit publicly that they are totally unprotected is often too bitter to endure."[3] An exception to the rule was women who accepted charity on behalf of their children and used the breadlines as takeout counters, carrying home pails of soup or stew for the family table. The growing number of business girls, on the other hand, preferred to disappear from the public eye and somehow fend for themselves.

As the winter of 1930 to 1931 unfolded, the fate of these women became one of the Depression's early puzzles. The left-wing journalist Meridel Le Sueur spoke from experience when she wrote a 1932 story on exactly this topic. "It is one of the great mysteries of the city," Le Sueur began,

> *where women go when they are out of work and hungry. There are not many women in the bread lines. . . . Yet there must be as many women out of jobs in cities and suffering extreme poverty as there are men. What happens to them? Where do they go? . . . I've lived in cities for many months broke, without help, too timid to get in bread lines. I've known many women to live like this until they simply faint on the street from privations, without saying a word to anyone.*[4]

For these women, hunger was a supremely private affliction. Rather than joining the lines, they banished themselves to shared apartments and boardinghouses and stayed put, "living on a cracker a day" as long as their rent held out. Stories in the popular press introduced these invisible women to the reading public, and before too long Hollywood versions of unemployed working girls became the new stars of Depression-era movie houses. In the Busby Berkeley extravaganza *Gold Diggers of 1933*, three exceptionally plucky young women, in this case out-of work chorus girls, share a single bedroom in a cheap Manhattan apartment.

Behind on their rent, and with their best clothes in hock, the girls start their day by pilfering a bottle of milk from a neighbor's windowsill, joking that if the wolf actually appeared at their door, they would eat him.

Through the winter of 1930 to 1931, the city's private charities continued to run on the highest gear, their expanded activities paid for mainly by the people of New York. Signs of progress, however, were elusive. No amount of charitable help, it appeared, could alleviate a quickly deteriorating situation. In fact, it began to seem that charity was part of the problem, and before the winter was half over, signs of a shift in perspective had started to surface. In January 1931, in a departure from the sympathetic treatment once reserved for the topic, the *New York Evening Post* ran a four-part story exposing the folly of the breadlines, the city's

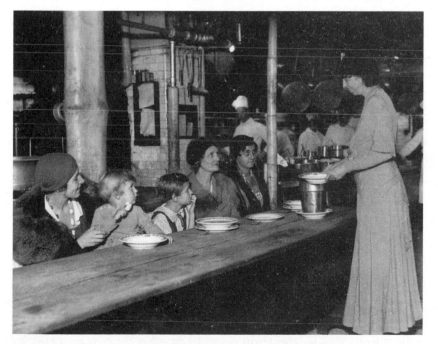

*Eleanor Roosevelt, then wife of the president-elect, serves soup to women and children in the kitchen of a New York restaurant, 1932.* (Everett Historical Collection, Alamy Stock Photo)

most visible form of charity. According to the *Post*, the problems began with the city's excessive number of breadlines. An open invitation to jobless men from across the United States, the sheer bounty of free food available in New York was turning the great metropolis into a public feeding station. To make matters worse, the new arrivals were capable freeloaders, quickly learning the ins and outs of the local food charities for the purpose of exploiting them. And the breadlines were eminently exploitable. With each line operating at different hours and no record of who received what, it was possible for a man to eat in as many as eight lines in a single day, his only limitation "the capacity of his stomach."[5] In between meals, the men panhandled, dozed, foraged for cigarettes, or applied for a new suit at one of the city's free clothing depots. The one activity they ran from was work, though in fact it was available to them. To help the jobless earn money, a number of breadlines offered short work stints splitting logs on charity woodlots. Their material needs met, however, the out-of-towners had no use for the woodpile, evidence that they were unworthy of help in the first place.

With uncanny precision, the *Post* series echoed turn-of-the-century arguments about the consequences of "indiscriminate charity." That the same charges could surface now, in the thick of so much adversity, showed the tenacity of America's ambivalence toward material relief in general, and food relief in particular. That ambivalence extended to the breadline's harshest critics, the city's social workers. Welfare professionals with a long-standing aversion to food charity, social workers condemned the breadlines as relief of the most haphazard and temporary variety, not much different from standing on a street corner and handing out nickels. The people who ran the breadlines, moreover, made no attempt to learn the first thing about the men they were trying to help, or to offer any form of "service" or counseling. The cause of more harm than good, the breadlines were humiliating and demoralizing and encouraged dependence, depriving able-bodied men of the impulse to fend for themselves. Social workers were adamant. Breadlines were the work of fumbling amateurs and "should be abolished entirely; if necessary by legal enactment." But the breadlines posed another kind of danger as well. The great swirl of publicity that surrounded them, the flurry of newspaper stories, photographs, and newsreels, diverted both attention and dollars away from other forms of relief, including those best suited to families, among the Depression's less publicized casualties.

---

THE BREADLINES, IT turned out, were a passing aberration that began to fade with the return of warm weather. Before 1931 was over, the city had forced most of them to close, allowing only a handful of the larger charities to continue their work. Likewise, the police department's mendicant squad had redoubled its efforts to clear out the army of panhandlers who had recently colonized New York, erasing another sign of distress. With the streets restored to order, it was reasonable to imagine that the city was recovering and would soon snap back to its former self.

People who made their living working with the poor, however, were confronted with evidence to the contrary. The Welfare Council of New York City was formed in 1925 to coordinate and advise the city's numerous charities. These were the boom years, at least for Wall Street, but social workers had already begun to notice creeping unemployment, the consequences of a changing American workplace. The present depression, in their eyes, was really one point along a continuum. By the fall of 1930, however, it was clear to social workers that the economic crises gripping urban America had reached historic dimensions and should be documented, now, while impressions were still vivid. With that in mind, the Welfare Council compiled *An Impressionistic View of the Winter of 1930–31 in New York City*, observations collected from hundreds of social workers and visiting nurses, distilled into a single volume by Lillian Brandt, a social worker and noted historian of her profession.[6]

*An Impressionistic View* describes the effects of unemployment on jobless New Yorkers, many of whom had never before turned to charities. Among the new applicants were

> *able bodied men of skill and good standing in well-paid seasonal occupations . . . musicians whose chances of employment had been taken away by the sound pictures; skilled cigar-makers for whose skill there was no market because of cigarettes and cigarette-making machines; waiters who had become superfluous because of the popularity of cafeterias; piano cabinet-makers and polishers, cap-makers, jewelers and others suffering from changes in taste and fashion. . . . There were young married men from families which had been under the care of social agencies when they were small children, but who had themselves been entirely self-supporting for ten or fifteen years. There were accountants, stock-and-bond salesmen, high-grade clerical workers; clothing manufacturers, contractors, and others who had been in business for themselves.*[7]

This diverse collection of individuals made up the ranks of the New Poor, whose single most pressing need was sufficient food for the family table. The public nurses and social workers who served the New Poor saw at close range how eating habits had deteriorated. People ate whatever they could get:

> *inferior qualities of food and less of it; less milk; loose milk instead of bottled milk, coffee for children who previously drank milk, less fruit and vegetables, no eggs; meat once a week or not at all when the custom had been to have it once a day; in short, a transformation of the abundant variety characteristic of the*

*diet of even the poor in New York City into a monotonous fare*
*consisting largely of starches and sugars.*[8]

For the nurses who contributed to the study, the health consequences of such limited fare were already visible. Inadequate food
was responsible for more sickness, longer convalescences, and an
all-around lack of vitality, starting with a loss of "pep" and building to reported cases of physical collapse.

Reluctant but growing awareness of malnourished New Yorkers was the cause for an experiment in mass feeding that combined
private money with the public machinery of city government. In
the fall of 1930, standing before an audience of his thirty-seven
commissioners, one for each municipal department, Mayor
Jimmy Walker announced his plans to help families affected
by the Depression. To carry them through the coming winter,
Walker would engage the city's various departments to create the
Mayor's Committee on Unemployment, a makeshift relief agency
that took existing structures of government and repurposed them,
supplying families with fuel, clothing, and, most important, food.
To pay for all that emergency help, the mayor would tap the city's
125,000 municipal workers, asking that they each donate 1 percent
of their monthly salaries to a special emergency fund. For any man
in the room who somehow mistook the committee for a form of
charity—a word that trailed a long list of negative associations—
the mayor offered stern correction. This was *not* a charity, he told
them, but a wholesome example of neighbor helping neighbor, exactly the kind of relief advocated by President Hoover.

The foot soldiers of Walker's experiment were the police, their
first order of business a citywide canvass of the unemployed. In the
final week of October 1930, officers in all seventy-two of the city's
precincts engaged in a door-to-door survey, compiling a master
list of families that could no longer provide for themselves. Based
on the officers' count, supplies purchased by the Department of

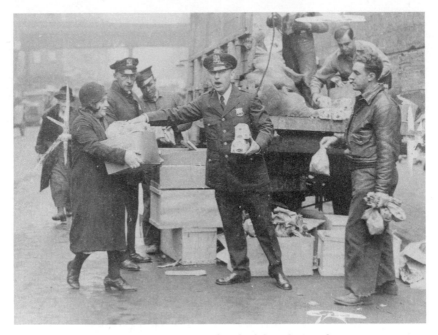

*New York City police precincts were used as food distribution depots, 1930.* (Library of Congress, LC-USZ62-115090)

Markets were delivered to precinct station houses by an armada of trucks courtesy of the Department of Sanitation. Distributions began on a wet November morning with the now familiar sight of food lines, only in this case they led to neighborhood police stations, the city's newest food relief depots. A combination of rain and the long wait was enough to drive away some of the crowd, but those who persevered were rewarded with a forty-pound quota of groceries, enough food to sustain a family of four for a week. The exact contents varied some from one week to the next, but typically included

> *20 pounds potatoes*
> *2 pounds beans*
> *2 pounds rice*
> *2 pounds macaroni*

*2 pounds onion*

*4 pounds cabbage*

*4 pounds turnips*

*8 pounds carrots*

*2 pounds sugar*

*1 pound coffee*

*1 pound evaporated milk*

*2 pounds canned tomatoes*[9]

On Thanksgiving and Christmas, the quotas were supplemented by a holiday fowl, and for Passover, Jewish New Yorkers received a four-pound ration of matzo.

The mayor's weekly distributions were an early example of the Depression's countless emergency diets, temporary strategies for answering the body's basic nutritional needs at the lowest possible cost. Like other emergency diets, it worked according to Atwater's principle of substitution, the idea that one food could be safely swapped out for a cheaper alternative, but only if it delivered the same nourishment or "food value." When he looked at a carrot or an onion or a lamb chop, Atwater saw a nutrient delivery system, a kind of edible apparatus for which taste, form, and texture were incidental qualities. Two foods that shared the same nutritional profile were as good as identical and therefore interchangeable, a single cheap food standing in for an entire food group. In substitution, Atwater saw nothing less than a means for improving the lives of American wage earners. The many dissatisfactions that beset the working class were, according to Atwater, the direct product of uninformed and excessive food spending. Substitution, a science-based approach to food selection, allowed people of limited means to free up money normally spent on groceries for other, more rewarding though unspecified uses. Among the foods on Atwater's "expendable" list were eggs, butter, chicken, meat, and fish. Fruits and green vegetables, though commendable as a source of bulk, were likewise unnecessary, their consumption discouraged. Condiments and seasonings (Atwater called them "food adjuncts") inflamed the appetite, leading to overconsumption, another form of waste, and were therefore to be avoided.

His food budget now appropriately trimmed, the worker was left with unadorned potatoes, cabbage, turnips, dried peas, and assorted cereals, the cheapest available sources of both energy and protein. The New York quotas paid tribute to the sturdy, utilitarian foods recommended by Atwater as replacements for more expensive fare. The cooking instructions that came with the quotas were equally Atwater-esque. On the premise that nourishing food should also be "plain," the city provided homemakers with instructions to wring the most nutrients from the accompanying ingredients while ensuring the utmost in culinary simplicity:

> *All vegetables should be thoroughly washed, pared and cooked in enough salted boiling water to cover. Cook with cover on the pot and until tender. Save water that vegetables are cooked in for soup stock.*
>
> *Dried beans are to be soaked in cold water over night. In the morning cover with fresh water, heat slowly and cook until skin will burst.*
>
> *Macaroni—cook in salted boiling water until tender. Drain water, then rinse off with cold water.*
>
> *Vegetable Soup—potatoes, onions, cabbage, turnips, beans and barley.*
>
> *Stock for soup can be made from the vegetables that they are cooked in.*
>
> *Beans—plain—or cooked with onions and tomatoes.*
>
> *Macaroni—plain—or cooked with onions and tomatoes.*
>
> *Cabbage, carrots and onions, raw sliced or boiled.*
>
> *Turnips—plain—cooked or mashed with potatoes.*[10]

Homemakers in need of additional guidance could also tune in to daily radio classes on WNYC, the city's radio station, which covered such topics as cooking with leftovers, meat substitutes, and food values in relation to cost.

———

JUST WEEKS INTO the 1930 school year, teachers across the city began to notice unusual attendance patterns, more children missing from the classroom and for longer periods than in normal years. As always, if a child skipped more than three days of school, the case required review by the Bureau of Attendance, the law enforcement arm of the Board of Education. Following established protocol, attendance officers were sent to students' homes to check on their whereabouts and, if warranted, to impose the appropriate punishment. When they arrived, however, instead of truants they found children barred from school by lack of adequate food and clothing.

Those officers became the unlikely heroes of a "vast benevolent movement" in which schools were transformed into emergency assistance centers. Organized along the same lines as the grocery distributions, the School Relief Fund was a joint production between city government and the people of New York, in this case the Board of Education employees whose monthly contributions bankrolled the fund. Those same employees doubled as impromptu relief workers. In their classrooms, teachers kept an eye open for children who looked to be in need of clothing, seemed unusually distracted, or tired too quickly, engaging them in "delicate and diplomatic" inquiry about conditions at home. Where it seemed that help was called for, the child was reported to one of the city's 340 attendance officers. If a home visit confirmed pressing need, relief was given on the spot, beginning in many cases with the students' feet. Equipped with sizing charts, officers took the children's measurements and returned later with new, properly fitting shoes, a transaction repeated in tens of thousands of households. By the end of December, the school system had purchased and delivered 28,378 pairs of sturdy, durable shoes "calculated to see their possessors through the Winter."[11] New shoes, however, were of limited value to children who were too undernourished to concentrate and, more seriously, too weak to attend school at all. Feeding those children became the schools' next mission.

The idea that city schools were in any way obliged to nourish their students came of age at the turn of the century with the School Lunch Movement, a cause that merged Progressive politics with the budding science of nutrition. Convinced that a poor diet was "the prime and most fruitful cause of mental dulness and its attendant evils," lunch reformers campaigned to provide impoverished children with the food they needed to learn.[12] New York's first lunch program was launched by concerned citizens and taken over by the Board of Education in 1920. Under the direction of the Department of Homemaking, school lunches were cooked in central kitchens in the city's two main tenement districts, one on the Lower East Side under the Williamsburg Bridge, the second in East Harlem, and trucked to nearby schools in insulated containers. By 1930, however, the problem of childhood hunger had overflowed the old tenement neighborhoods, an eventuality for which schools were utterly unprepared.

To catch up with the present reality, the Department of Homemaking patched together an expanded lunch program. Wherever needed, homemaking instructors were pressed into service, their classrooms converted into working kitchens staffed by student cooks. (Morning classes were used to prepare that day's lunch, while afternoons were devoted to the next day's dessert.) In schools that had no kitchens, stoves were installed in basements or gymnasiums. Lunch counters were created from wooden planks supported by old desks, the surfaces covered in brightly colored oilcloth. Emergency menus and recipes were created and disseminated to all of these satellite lunchrooms, each of them patrolled by an experienced teacher of homemaking to ensure uniform standards.

Orchestrating this surge of activity was the director of homemaking for the New York school system. Having taught in the public schools since 1906, Martha Westfall was clearly a woman of ample experience. Even so, the job was daunting. "Each day," she confessed,

> *brings its discouragements and what seem to be insurmountable obstacles. But every morning means a new day and yesterday's worries are cleared away to make way for fresh ones. Even the weather seems to conspire against the lunches, and when perfectly good rice pudding leaves the kitchen only to sour on the way, and when innocent beans decide to ferment in the humid atmosphere, or when the cook's back is turned and the soup burns, then problems of international importance seem but trifles in comparison with the troubles of those responsible for feeding hundreds of hungry children.*[13]

To imagine that lives depended on the school kitchen was no delusion of grandeur. For many students, lunch was their only meal of the day; parents counted on it, not only for the sake of the child, but with one meal covered by the lunchroom, more food was left for the rest of the family. Alternately, children saved food from their lunch trays to take home to parents, brothers, and sisters. Anything transportable was slipped into trouser pockets, though supervisors also caught one determined boy filling a handkerchief with chocolate pudding. Another was observed scraping the butter from his bread to stash away for his mother.[14] (For the record, despite workplace pressures, Westfall stayed at her post for the duration of the Depression and continued in her job for most of World War II as well.)

The school lunch diet reflected what experts of the day declared nutritionally essential foods for children. At the center of the diet there was milk. As a source of protein for building muscles, minerals for the health of teeth and bones, vitamins to protect the body from disease, and sugars and fats to give it energy, milk was believed to provide the very best building blocks for construction and upkeep of the "human house." Accordingly, Westfall introduced milk into the substance of every meal. Creamed soups, creamed vegetables, puddings, custards, and cocoa were all lunchtime staples, and this was in addition to the half pint of milk served to each child as a beverage. The following is one of Westfall's four rotating menus:

### MONDAY

*Cocoa*

*Tomato puree*

*Succotash*

*Cheese sandwich*

*Fresh or stewed fruit*

### TUESDAY

*Pea soup (without milk)*

*Italian spaghetti with onion and*
*    tomato sauce*

*White rolls, buttered*

*Chocolate pudding, served with milk*

### WEDNESDAY

*Tomato macaroni soup (thickened*
*    with farina)*

*Baked salmon or creamed Friday*
*    salmon*

*Buttered graham roll*
*Rich custard pudding*

### THURSDAY
*Vegetable soup with rice*
*Creamed lima beans*
*Whole wheat bread and butter*
    *sandwich*
*Stewed or fresh fruit or fruit gelatin*
    *or fruit salad*

### FRIDAY
*Lima bean and barley soup*
*Jam or fish sandwich, whole wheat*
    *bread*
*Creamed carrots with peas or creamed*
    *cabbage or mashed turnips*
*Vanilla cornstarch pudding, chocolate*
    *sauce*[15]

To further guarantee adequate milk consumption (a quart per day was ideal, but a pint was acceptable), milk and crackers were served as snacks at recess.

From the start, school lunch was thought to serve a double purpose: it both nourished and enlightened. Accordingly, the school lunchroom was simultaneously a dining facility and a teaching forum, a "laboratory from which to disseminate food knowledge." The hugely expanded lunch program necessitated by the Depression provided a rare teaching opportunity, and educators seized the moment, impassioned by the belief that the need for food knowledge had never been greater. In the lunchroom, the menu was its own curriculum, an example of how children were supposed to eat. Its content, however, was reinforced throughout the school day. In English class, children wrote compositions on one or another aspect of nutrition, while for art they drew nutrition-inspired posters that were hung on school walls, persistent reminders of cardinal food facts. In music class, nutritional information was expressed in song, an especially effective teaching method, as facts put to music "sink deep in minds of children."[16]

Alongside fact-based instruction, lunches tutored children in the more subjective realm of taste. In America's most diverse city, a babel of gastronomic traditions, school lunchrooms introduced a common culinary language—in this case the mild, "easily digested" fare endorsed by home economists. Getting children, particularly immigrant children, to eat it required gentle indoctrination on the part of lunchroom teachers, a task they were fully prepared to take on. Carefully recording each child's nationality, teachers tracked which foods were willingly consumed and which were rejected. Reluctant eaters received patient encouragement, never reprimands. When introducing new foods, teachers relied on the power of repetition to make the strange seem more familiar. In the most stubborn cases, special measures were taken. Family members were called in to the lunchroom to provide added coaxing, or, conversely, food was sent home with the child. In the end, efforts to retrain young taste buds were a shining success. As a direct result of school lunches, children of diverse national backgrounds learned to eat and enjoy items like Boston baked beans and cornstarch pudding, "foods found in the ordinary American dietary," which initially they had refused to even taste.[17] Unexpectedly, some food preferences cut across ethnic divisions. Regardless of ethnicity, all children seemed to appreciate buttered white bread and canned peaches. Conversely, foods disliked by the majority of students were lettuce and anything cooked in white sauce.

"IF THE STORY of New York City's fight against human misery during this depression is ever written, the public school teachers will be found to have contributed one of the finest chapters of it."[18] So began one of many public expressions of gratitude for the guardians of New York schoolkids. A voice of dissent came from the welfare experts who observed the teachers in action and found them wanting, their critique laid out in the pages of Brandt's *Impressionistic View*:

> Because of inexperience in social work, teachers and principals were "solicitous," "over-solicitous," "too enthusiastic," "sentimental," "over protective. . . ." They did not understand the "deeper social aspects." Their methods were "haphazard" and they "tended to apply themselves to the wrong angle of many situations."[19]

Solicitous one minute, a beat later they were capable of blunt insensitivity, asking by a show of hands which children had a father out of work and announcing to the class where that parent should go for help. Confirmation of the fact that they were unprepared, however, was the teachers' inability to effectively size up their welfare clients. In the absence of well-honed detective skills—a must for any social worker—school employees fell into the dreaded trap of indiscriminate giving, arbitrarily handing out aid both to people in real need and to those who could manage on their own.

As agents of food charity, the police were even more roundly criticized, beginning with the rations they provided: "The food itself was not enough for families of large size. . . . It did not meet the needs of small children or convalescents or pregnant women or nursing mothers. It was not adapted to the food habits of the different nationalities," and among those who relied on it exclusively, it was responsible for multiple cases of "gastric disturbance."[20] What's more, the department's very public method of food distribution was "inconsiderate and demoralizing," with people standing for hours in the cold and rain in plain sight of their neighbors, and with mothers and children forced to lug home forty-pound cartons containing little more than potatoes, a special hardship in "rural boroughs" where distances were longer.

It was a point of fact among social workers that charity presented certain well-known psychological risks. The winter of 1930 to 1931 showed that industrious, well-adjusted Americans were just as susceptible as anyone else. Humiliation inflicted on jobless New Yorkers by the various improvised charities told the story in a nutshell. A crash course in emergency relief, the winter also convinced social workers of their own inadequacies. The New Poor were different from the kinds of people who normally applied to the charities; they therefore required a new approach. Job hunting was its own degrading ordeal, but for people who had always imagined themselves immune to poverty, the decision to go to the charities was a final admission of personal failure. Once the plunge was taken, however, it quickly became a habit, and people who had never imagined themselves reliant on anyone lapsed into "a position of dependence."[21] As the winter progressed, social workers came to the uncomfortable realization that they were adding to the psychological wreckage, and that it was time for everyone to try something new.

# Chapter 4

———◦•◦———

THE STATE OF Iowa, President Hoover's beloved birthplace, was a land of rich soil, cornfields that stretched to the sky every summer, and fat hogs in every farmyard. In October 1929, Iowans paid only brief attention to news of the Wall Street crash that was splashed across the front pages. Rumors circulated about which local businessmen in cities like Des Moines had dabbled too much in the market and lost everything, but the general consensus was that the stock market decline might even help Iowa. Business leaders predicted that money that had previously gone to Wall Street would now be deposited in local banks and invested in Iowa businesses. Local newspapers ran articles predicting a rosy future for rural America:

> *The sun is always shining on business somewhere. The industrial east is clouded but the agricultural west seems to be in for a spell of fair weather. It appears that the farmers were very little hurt by the stock market crash. Most of the damage was done in the large cities of the country and the thickly settled industrial areas of the east. As we travel from east to west we cannot help but notice a more optimistic feeling as we go. To be sure, grain prices slumped with stocks at first, but have since made a good recovery. Total farm incomes for 1929 will be at least as large as in 1928 and may be larger. Unquestionably,*

*as between the various sectors of our population, the farmers
are now in the preferred position.*[1]

The top banker in Muscatine, Iowa, told the Associated Press
that the forecast for local farms was "more promising than it has
been at any time since the slump of 1921," while a Muscatine
farmer predicted better profits from the all-important hog industry: "Corn is reasonably cheap. The hog crop is short for the
coming year which leads to expectation of higher prices. Present
hog prices are above those of a year ago."[2] Like the rest of rural
America, Iowa had been mired in an agricultural depression for
most of a decade. Prices for corn, hogs, wheat, beef, cabbages, and
apples couldn't fall much lower and therefore had to go up. That,
of course, was incorrect.

By early 1930, the prices for all major agricultural commodities,
including fruits, grains, vegetables, and livestock, had begun to
drop. The cause of this slide was steadily decreasing demand for
farm products, in both the United States and overseas markets.
The price of corn on the Chicago commodity exchange fell from
about a dollar a bushel in late 1929 to less than a quarter by mid-
1932. This should have been good for Iowa's hog farmers, because
feeding livestock was that much less expensive, but hog prices also
dropped by more than 50 percent. It didn't pay to feed the pigs,
let alone take them to market. Deflation hit nearly every agricultural region of the United States. During the 1920s, farmers
had plowed up a million acres of virgin western Kansas lands and
planted mile after mile of hard winter wheat. Aided by a stretch of
abundant rainfall, they increased production every year, earning
about $1.25 a bushel in 1927. That price had dropped to sixty-three
cents a bushel by 1930, yet Kansas farmers remained optimistic
and planted even more wheat. The following spring, they enjoyed
a record crop, but received only thirty-three cents a bushel, not
enough to cover production costs. The farmers knew in theory

that the only way to push up prices was to cut production, but it was difficult to swallow a temporary loss of income when they had invested everything in their land and farm equipment and had no savings to tide them over. Nevertheless, in April 1931, the United States Wheat Growers Union declared a strike: They would neither sell nor plant any wheat until the price reached a dollar a bushel. Kansas farmers couldn't imagine how their situation could get even worse. (Later that summer, the rains stopped falling, and hot and dusty winds began to blow.)

The twin problems of deflation and decreasing demand struck not only farms concentrating on one or two commodities but even those producing diverse crops. Violet Krall grew up on her family's twenty-acre truck farm just outside Milwaukee. Descended from German immigrants, her parents grew vegetables and kept cows, pigs, and a flock of chickens. They sold their vegetables, as well as flowers, eggs, butter, buttermilk, bacon, and sausages, at the downtown Milwaukee wholesale market, where their customers were mostly city grocery stores and restaurants. Then the Depression hit, and suddenly their buyers disappeared:

> *I was seven or eight at the time. One of my brothers and I prepared green onions for the market, involving washing all the dirt off the onions and bunching them. That day when my father returned from the market, he first stopped and threw the unsold onions on the manure pile—all he had taken to the market except two bunches. I wanted to cry. All that work, and no one wanted to buy them.*

Violet's father decided to drop his stall at the market and build up a truck route, going door to door through Milwaukee's more affluent neighborhoods to sell his produce. His new business kept the family alive, although there were still many days when the farm produced more than customers would buy:

*The chickens did not know there was a Depression and would very often lay more eggs than would meet the needs of our customers and our own, so we ate a lot of eggs. I took my lunch to school and was joined by classmates who lived at a distance too great to allow them to go home for lunch. Once, as I was beginning to eat my egg salad sandwich, the girl in the seat next to mine said, "You must be rich." I asked her why she said that, and she said that they could not afford eggs. I offered to trade with her—her peanut butter and jelly sandwich for my egg salad. I thought it was a good trade, since we did not have enough cash to buy peanut butter. What a treat![3]*

The market economy's retreat affected different parts of rural America in different ways. In Iowa, corn and hogs were mainstays of the local economy. The steep drop in prices was a grievous blow to nearly every farm family. Near their nadir in early 1931, a farmer named Arthur Johnson composed a poem called "Tough Going":

> *The price of feed is high,*
> *Eggs are sold for naught;*
> *But the market seems to take delight*
> *And oleo is being bought.*
>
> *There is a depression going on,*
> *That causes furrows in the brow*
> *Wheat and corn are sold as gifts,*
> *But that is old news now.*
>
> *The farmer raises twice as much*
> *As he did some years ago;*
> *The old plow doesn't scour well,*
> *In being twice as low.*

*The farmer lives a storm-tossed life,*
*Like a rowboat in the sea*
*He's up and down, and twirled about,*
*But he still can smile, by Gee!*[4]

Iowa farmers could smile because they lived in a state blessed by fertile soil, and if they were lucky, they didn't owe money to the bank or a mortgage company. They still had their farms. Most Iowa farm families still lived largely as their parents and grandparents had, plowing their fields with horse or ox teams. Their homes lacked electricity, running water, and modern appliances. They relied on corn and hogs for a cash income, but they still grew most of what they ate. When the Depression hit, they retreated from the larger economy to their farms and local communities, finding any means of "making do."

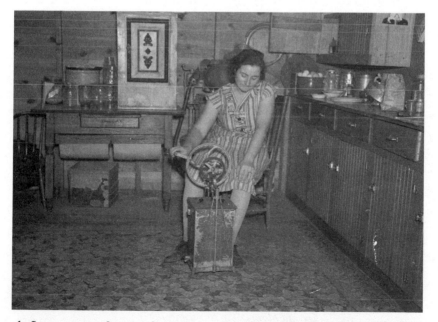

*An Iowa woman churning butter in a well-appointed farmhouse kitchen.* (Russell Lee photographer, Farm Security Administration Collection, Library of Congress, LC-DIG-fsa-8b30017)

For most farm families, it was easy to fall back on nineteenth-century cycles of subsistence farming, from the early spring gathering of wild greens to the late autumn hog butchering. As the Depression worsened, however, farmers were also eager to adopt any modern farming techniques that might help them survive. The local farm extension agents, employed by the state's department of agriculture, were full of the latest ideas on soil science and increasing yields, but their suggestions were of little value if there was no market for farm products. It was the home extension agents, all of them women and also on the state payroll, who were far more influential in helping farm families survive the economic downturn. Most of these women were trained as home economists, full of information on the science of cooking, sewing, and cleaning, with an emphasis on modern technology, hygiene, and affordability. The home agent assigned to each district would visit farmhouses to pass out pamphlets, give lectures in town, and convene regular meetings of the local homemakers' club. The topics at these events were all eminently practical: how to make your own soap, sew children's dresses, weave a rug from old rags, bake Christmas pies, get grease stains out of your husband's Sunday trousers, and so on. At a time when they had little money to buy ingredients at the local store, many women avidly attended discussions on how to produce more food at home.

Most Iowa farms already had gardens; now they were expanded to cover as much ground as the housewife and her children could hoe. To encourage this trend, in late 1931 the United States Department of Agriculture issued a bulletin titled "The Farm Garden," which informed farmers that a well-maintained half-acre garden could supply vegetables with a market value of $100 to $150. The traditional garden crops included corn, potatoes, onions, cabbages, turnips, parsnips, lettuce, cucumbers, and peas. Now the government encouraged farmers to also grow more leafy vegetables, such as spinach and chard, for their nutritional value. In Iowa's climate zone, farmhouse gardens could produce fresh vegetables for only five or six months of the year. Luckily, home extension agents were full of ideas on how they could be preserved for the long, cold winters. These included various cellaring methods for potatoes and onions, special pits to hold cabbages, turnips, and beets, and, most important, canning.

The technology to preserve food in hermetically sealed glass jars or metal containers had been around for more than a century, but it hadn't been widely adopted for home use until the food conservation drive during World War I. Now, at the urging of home extension agents, there was a sudden run on canning jars and lids. In southern Illinois, where farmers were particularly desperate, they hoped to can a bumper fruit crop: "In August and September the peach trees were loaded down with beautiful fruit, and the people were being urged to can as much as possible. But on every hand one heard the cry, 'We have no cans!'"[5] From the garden, vegetables were taken into the kitchen, usually during the hottest days of the summer, where the housewife spent days slaving over a red-hot stove to preserve her bounty for the winter. There was no question that this effort was worth it. One Iowa woman wrote to a farm journal: "I'm canning everything in sight. No matter what comes, *we're going to eat!*"[6]

Home extension agents were just one source of information on how best to ride out the Depression; farm women also turned to local newspapers, women's magazines, farm journals, and if they were lucky enough to have electricity, the radio. Although broadcast radio was barely a decade old, its signals already covered a broad swath of rural America. Broadcasters soon discovered that they had a captive audience in the multitudes of farm women who were occupied with daily chores at home while their husbands worked in the fields. Big food manufacturers began to sponsor homemaking shows, usually heavy on recipes and running in the morning hours (the precursor to daytime television). The fictional character of Betty Crocker was invented by one of the flour companies that later became part of General Mills. In 1924, "Betty Crocker" debuted as the narrator of a radio cooking school show, running twice a week at 10:30 a.m.; by 1930 it was heard over forty-three stations nationwide.

Not to be outdone, in 1926 the U.S. Department of Agriculture's farm radio service debuted a five-day-a-week show called *Housekeepers' Chat* hosted by "Aunt Sammy" (presumably some sort of consort to Uncle Sam). On the show, Aunt Sammy sat at the center of a large, somewhat inept family who regularly came to her with questions on everything from how to prepare a Thanksgiving pie to why children needed sunbaths. In reality, she was a folksy vehicle for the USDA's Bureau of Home Economics to disseminate its expert advice on "nutrition, meal-planning, cooking, clothing, health, house furnishing, gardening, and other kindred subjects."[7] The fifteen-minute scripts were prepared in Washington and sent to dozens of stations across the country to be read by each station's own "Aunt Sammy" in the local accent and with her own embellishments. The formula was an instant success; the first four months of the show generated 25,000 letters from homemakers seeking advice. Many of those letters asked for cooking advice, so in 1927 the Bureau of Home Economics published its first edition of *Aunt Sammy's Radio Recipes*, given free to anyone who requested a copy. By 1931, the show was a regular feature on well over a hundred stations nationwide, and many thousands of copies of the cookbook had been distributed, primarily to the show's rural listeners.

Like most home economists, the experts behind *Housekeepers' Chat* believed in the importance of simple, nutritious, and inexpensive dishes. As conditions in rural America deteriorated, they increased the emphasis on preparing budget meals. A December 1931 show titled "An Inexpensive Christmas Menu" began: "A less expensive dinner for a thrifty Christmas can be just as good and just as Christmasy as one planned with all the frills and expensive items of food."[8] Its recipes included a baked ham and, in lieu of a traditional plum pudding, a chocolate gelatin made with raisins, dates, nuts, and currants. A show titled "Low Cost Meals" focused on the many people who needed help "planning well-balanced healthful diets for families with limited incomes." After pointing out the dangers of the staple "meat-potato-pie-and-pancake" rural diet, Aunt Sammy turned to the bureau's experts for a meal plan based on the latest nutritional science:

> *They suggest that when there is little money to spend for food, the diet should be built around the grain products and milk, with enough vegetables and fruits to supply the necessary additional vitamins and minerals. Lean meat, fish, poultry and eggs, which are more expensive, should be used sparingly. The fruits and vegetables should be those that are in season and where possible, less expensive in price. Tomatoes, cabbage, carrots and onions are all inexpensive vegetables and well worth using frequently for family meals.*[9]

The menu for the show included shredded string beans cooked with leftover pork, potato salad, stewed prunes and apricots for dessert, and oatmeal cookies. During long rural winters, Aunt Sammy also suggested that women grow parsley plants on kitchen windowsills and use the leaves to brighten up their dishes (and help their families avoid seasonal vitamin deficiencies).

While housewives, particularly in the Midwest, avidly joined extension clubs and consumed home economics information, their husbands found their own, informal ways to keep their farms afloat. Although they, and their entire communities, were cash-poor, they still grew crops that someone else might want. From the most isolated rural farms to suburban truck gardens,

Depression-era farmers rediscovered the barter economy that had sustained their frontier ancestors. If a farmer needed, say, barn repairs or house painting, he might offer a carpenter or painter a bushel of potatoes or a pair of chickens for the work. The most popular center for the new barter economy was the country store. One store owner in the tiny, impoverished town of Prosperity, Arkansas, told a journalist: "At least a third of my business is done in barter. I take herbs, hides, poultry, eggs, cream and butter, sometimes strawberries, potatoes, fruit and corn in exchange for store goods."[10] In return, the farmer could purchase tobacco, sugar, coffee, soda crackers, wheat flour, canned goods, cooking utensils, and a wide variety of non-food wares. Although some farmers resisted, bartering quickly became a way of life:

> *Swapping gets in a person's blood after staying in the country awhile. One day I told Buddy to take some eggs to the store and swap them for some salt, coffee, and sugar. That nearly killed him; he was ashamed to let the storekeeper know we didn't have the money to buy what he needed. I explained how thankful he ought to be that we had something to swap. Even after all I said, he went away resentful, talking to the mule and hoping he'd fall and make him break every one of the eggs. Just to show he changed—six months later, he'd swap eggs for anything, even a ticket to a picture show.*[11]

In the wheat-growing region of western Kansas, farmers were broke, but store owners in nearby towns agreed to take wheat for their goods in lieu of cash, even at restaurants:

> *After paying for his meal in a café, a local landowner capped the climax by tipping the waitress in Marland a bushel of wheat. His meal cost him two bushels of wheat and two of oats. He*

*had just completed threshing both crops, with wheat at 25 cents a bushel and oats at 17½. Another landowner of Kay County, while threshing his wheat, took seven employees to town for luncheon, which cost him 50 cents a man, or a total of fifteen bushels of wheat.*[12]

Unfortunately, not everyone had enough crops for barter. In order to supplement what they had grown, they picked up sacks and went into nearby woods and fields to forage for wild foods. Sometimes these expeditions took foragers across property lines that had been largely ignored before the Depression. When Rowena May Pope was a child in northeastern Missouri, she and her siblings used to explore along railroad tracks and around pastures, looking for gooseberries:

> *One day after we had tramped for hours picking the sour little berries and our muslin flour sacks were nearly filled, we were surprised by a man carrying a rifle.*
>
> *He shouted, "Lay down those berries and get out of here!"*
>
> *We couldn't believe our eyes. We knew that man. He was the father of one of our schoolfriends. We responded, "You're only joking, right?"*
>
> *"No, I'm not joking," he answered firmly.*
>
> *We realized he was serious, so we put down our bags and trudged home.*[13]

Only the property owner and his family would enjoy gooseberry cobbler that evening.

In fact, the economic crisis greatly increased tensions, both social and personal, across Iowa and the rest of rural America. The rate of farm foreclosures skyrocketed, and with it rose the number of suicides and murders. To make ends meet, some Iowans turned to moonshining and running bootleg liquor or outright criminality. Teams of robbers ransacked small-town banks that had managed to ride out the downturn and raided farmhouses whose owners were rumored to have secret hoards of money. Nearly every farmer faced the problem of thievery. At night, or when families were in church on Sunday morning, thieves would steal milk off their porches, take whole hams hanging from the timbers of their smokehouses, and, most commonly of all, raid the chicken house. John Johnson, whose spread was outside Moravia, Iowa, was one of many farmers who slept with a shotgun beside themselves, ready to leap up and start blasting at the sound of irregular clucking in the barnyard:

> *It all happened something like this. Mrs. Johnson was sleeping on a porch at the rear of the house. About 1:30 she was aroused by a peculiar noise from the direction of the chicken house. Getting up, she went to the door in time to see a man round the corner of the chicken house and go inside. She immediately called Mr. Johnson, who, as soon as aroused, grabbed a shotgun and started for the chicken house. However, Mr. Thief evidently became alarmed and lost no time in leaving that vicinity. Mr. Johnson fired several times in the direction in which the thief was travelling but does not know whether or not he scored a hit.*[14]

The thief never was caught, escaping with thirty of the Johnsons' finest spring chickens. He was lucky; many chicken thieves were wounded or even killed while attempting to steal the birds.

As the barnyard crime wave rose, farmers urged a crackdown:

> *Of all the thieves the one most despised is the fellow who steals chickens. The expression "as low down as a chicken thief" carries with it the limit in condemnation, and no man who has the least atom of self-respect will ever be guilty of such*

*conduct as to merit the term "chicken thief" being applied to him. However, the stealing of poultry is growing to be a major industry and until courts and especially juries realize that the chicken thief must be rated as a major thief the stealing of chickens will continue.*[15]

However, no law could stop the desperation that drove people to crime, so thievery remained part of rural life throughout the Depression era.

For those who, through a combination of bad luck and the dire economy, had lost their farms and jobs, there was little government safety net in Iowa or other rural regions of the country. All that most counties offered was a poor farm. This was a facility, usually just outside the county seat, where paupers were housed in a farmhouse, usually a rambling, old wood-framed structure that was sustained by a large garden and a few cows, chickens, and hogs. The poor farm was reserved for "designated paupers," who were defined as "deserving poor" who couldn't work and had no family to support them, usually the aged, handicapped, and mentally ill. Traditionally, and by design, there was great shame in "going on the county." A popular poem called "Over the Hill to the Poor House" recounts the humiliation of a widow who was rejected by her children, one of whom sends her to the poorhouse:

> *So they have shirked and slighted me, an' shifted me about—*
> *So they have well nigh soured me, an' wore my old heart out;*
> *But still I've born up pretty well, an' wasn't much put down,*
> *Till Charley went to the poor-master, an' put me on the town!*
>
> *Over the hill to the poor-house—my child'rn dear, good-bye!*
> *Many a night I've watched you when only God was nigh;*
> *And God'll judge between us; but I will al'ays pray*
> *That you shall never suffer the half that I do to-day!*[16]

The quality of the poorhouses varied from county to county. The supervisors were nearly always untrained, and budgets ranged from reasonable to bare-bones. In some, residents lived relatively comfortable lives, while in others they were half-starved. The supervisor's salary and budget for house upkeep came out of the same pot; some unscrupulous operators discovered that the less they fed their charges, the more they could put into their own pockets. When the Depression hit, this antiquated system quickly came under strain.

As 1930 stretched into 1931, many able-bodied Iowans lost their farms and jobs and were unable to find work. The existing poor farm system was ill equipped to deal with this crisis. Poor farms were not meant to house able-bodied men and families with small children, and their supervisors had no idea how to feed the rapidly growing numbers of newly poor. Counties tried a variety of methods to cope, usually a combination of direct relief—giving food, fuel, and so on—and work relief. In Bremer County, Iowa, the board of supervisors reviewed every case and tried to put the men to work on town repair projects. If that wasn't possible, the needy were given scrip or vouchers to spend on food and other supplies at local stores. However, the rising number of jobless families quickly depleted the relief budget. In September 1930, Butler County had $10,000 in its relief fund; a year later it was $7,000 in debt. This work was supposed to be paid for by local taxes, but taxpayers were also feeling their own strains and beginning to resent those who received a "free ride" on their dollar. The Algona County board of supervisors, swamped with so many needy they couldn't investigate them all, decided to publish their names in order to "stem a tide of applications which has put the poor fund in the red and threatens to send it to new low depths."[17]

In Sioux County, where the names were still kept secret but everybody knew everybody else's business, a newspaper columnist opposed to handouts of food and money did his own investigation of the relief rolls:

*He finds many among them that are well posted on sports and the frills of life, but leave the job of making a living to the taxpayers. Fellows who perform gracefully behind the steering wheel, and have burned, and still burn the gas of joy to excess. He finds also the ex-bootlegger or the one still feebly functioning, and who refused honest labor when it was offered at every hand. One refused to work for $2.25 per day, and bragged about it. One able bodied young fellow was one of the first to have his car licensed. Another, not long from the land of the Dakotas, told his landlady "to go to h___" when she asked for the house rent. The county is paying for it now.[18]*

In the name of the taxpayer, he hoped that these "tax eaters" would take advantage of the coming corn-husking season and "sally forth to the fields at wages corresponding to the price of corn." He did not, however, mention whether he found any of the deserving poor on the rolls.

In response to the outcry caused by this column, the board made all relief applicants fill out a detailed form with questions like: Do you own a radio? Do you own a car? Do you spend any money for movies and entertainment? Did you plant a garden? How many bushels of potatoes do you have? The board gave aid in the form of scrip, which now could only be used to purchase the "necessities of life" at local stores: "flour, potatoes, navy beans, corn meal, oatmeal, coffee, tea, sugar, rice, yeast cakes, baking soda, pepper, matches, butter, lard, canned milk, laundry soap, prunes, syrup, tomatoes, canned peas, salmon, salt, vinegar, eggs, kerosene."[19] No one knew how long that aid would last, because the country poor fund had already spent $45,000 and was deeply in debt. Worse, farmers had reaped another bumper corn crop, keeping the prices low of not only corn but hogs. For the coming year, Iowa agricultural experts' best advice to farmers was to neither expand nor contract production, but just "sit tight" and hope for an economic upswing.

DURING THE 1930S, as in centuries past, the self-sustaining family farm remained the predominant unit of American agriculture in Iowa and elsewhere. However, farmers in some rural regions were increasingly devoting themselves to crop monocultures, from the potato fields of northern Maine to the Great Plains wheat fields and sprawling fruit and vegetable fields of California's Central Valley. Farms were increasingly becoming agribusinesses, each with professional managers and dozens or even hundreds of employees, all reliant on regional or national marketplaces to sell their product. By far the oldest and largest of these monocultures was found in the Cotton Belt, a vast swath of land distinctive for its rich soil, hot and steamy summers, and cool winters running from southern Virginia to East Texas.

The heart of this region was the Mississippi Delta, an alluvial plain that was covered with some of the darkest and richest farmland on earth and that bordered the seething, muddy river between Arkansas and Louisiana on the west and Mississippi on the east. Here, cotton was the main and in many places the only crop; the region's entire economy rose and fell with its wholesale price. Cotton farms were organized in plantations that covered as many as 40,000 acres and were often owned by corporations controlled by investors in New Orleans or even London. Although mechanization was coming to the Delta, most of the work was still done by mule team and by human labor—calloused hands swinging the hoe under the summer sun and picking the bolls at harvesttime.

Called tenant farmers, the men and women who tended the fields and harvested the cotton labored in a relationship clearly descended from that of master and slave in the pre–Civil War South, an annual contract replacing the master's deed of ownership. The majority of these farmers were black, although poor white laborers also worked the fields, particularly farther from the river. In either case, each tenant farmer family—father, mother, and children—agreed to tend twelve to twenty-four acres of cotton fields in return for a share of the harvest, as well as the use of fertilizer, mules, and meager living quarters. Perched in the middle of the cotton fields, these homes were sloppily built, two- or three-room shotgun shacks furnished with a few sticks of furniture (owned by the landlord) and wallboards covered with smoke-stained newspapers that did little to keep out the winter cold or summer mosquitoes. In the kitchen, the only equipment was a wood-fired stove, a table, a couple of chairs, and a few shelves. Water came from a well out in the yard. The poorest tenants, called sharecroppers, also had to rely on the plantation owner for food, which was credited against their share of the crop. The result of this system was that many tenant farmers were caught in a permanent web of debts. In the event of disagreement, black farmers could not turn to the courts, because they were controlled by the local white power structure and backed by Jim Crow laws enacted to keep blacks in their place. During World War I, when war industries desperate for workers offered blacks free tickets to cities like Pittsburgh and Detroit, white farmers enlisted local police to patrol railway stations and block them from embarking for the North. Whites also resorted to lynching and terrorism from groups like the Ku Klux Klan to keep blacks in line.

Food consumed by the tenant farmers was another relic of slave-era traditions. The main difference was that, in many cases, slaves were better fed. For seven or eight months a year, the farm owner provided his workers with a "plantation ration" of white flour, cornmeal, salt pork, and molasses—also known as the "three m" (meat, meal, and molasses) diet. At other times, they subsisted on hunting or fishing and on whatever they raised in their tiny gardens, if they were lucky enough to have one. By late winter, however, their cupboards contained only a small slab of salt pork, near-empty sacks of cornmeal, rice, and black-eyed

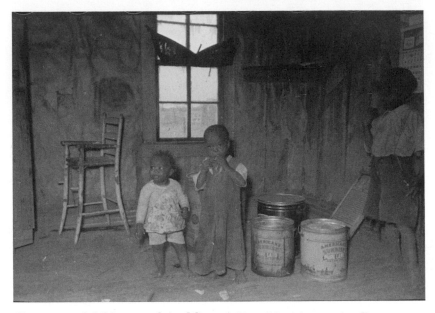

*Sharecroppers' children, southeast Missouri.* (Russell Lee photographer, Farm Security Administration Collection, Library of Congress, LC-DIG-fsa-8a22645)

peas, and a bit of coffee. Meals—only two a day—consisted of a monotonous round of rice, cornbread, and coffee for breakfast and then peas and cornbread for dinner. If they were lucky, farmers could add a bit of protein to the diet if they had laying chickens or by catching fish and trapping rabbits. Most of the time, however, all they did was tighten their belts and huddle around barely warm stoves, listening to the wind whistling through the cracks in the wallboards. As they waited for planting and the start of the new season's contracts, children grew hollow-eyed and listless and began to lose weight, while older folks suffered from indigestion, nervousness, and dizziness. Malnutrition diseases such as rickets and pellagra, also known as the "red flame," were common and potentially fatal. In March, however, they signed their contracts for the new season; the plantation owner handed out their ration of meat, meal, and molasses; and, like all farmers, they began to work with hope for the success of the year's crop. And it was generally agreed along the Delta that the spring of 1930 was uncommonly fine. The sun shone; the right amount of rain fell; and the landscape was green with row after row of cotton plants.

Just three years earlier, these same Delta fields had been a scene of devastation. Spurred by uncommonly heavy rains, in April 1927, the Mississippi River jumped the levees and flooded 27,000 square miles of farmland, including much of the Delta, killing well over two hundred people. The disaster was so severe that local governments were powerless to help. President Coolidge called in Herbert Hoover, then secretary of commerce, who led a massive operation to rescue, house, and feed flood victims. However, Hoover refused to spend federal funds on the relief effort. He followed the conservative tradition of presidents such as Grover Cleveland, who in 1887 rejected drought aid to Texas farmers: "The lesson should be constantly enforced that though the people support the Government, the Government should not support the people."[20]

In combating the 1927 flood, Hoover obeyed that directive, at least at first. An Iowa farm boy who had risen to fortune and position, Hoover firmly believed that rugged individualism was a central American virtue. To him, self-help and local voluntarism would be the backbone of the relief effort. However, he also had a pragmatic streak that identified a role for the federal government in helping combat the flood. He enlisted the American Red Cross, a quasi-governmental organization chartered by Congress, to plan and direct relief operations. During the worst of the crisis, Hoover also convinced the U.S. Army to distribute emergency rations, tents, and blankets directly to tens of thousands of refugees who were trapped on levees and in danger of starvation. The floodwaters eventually receded, leaving a fetid, muddy plain interspersed with ruined homes. Hoover marshaled state governments to rebuild roads and bridges and extend credit to local banks so they could give low-interest loans to farmers. The Red Cross gave cotton and vegetable seeds and farm implements to farmers so they could feed themselves and begin rehabilitating their land. Although Coolidge and Hoover never acknowledged it, in the end the federal government disbursed at least as much in disaster relief funds as was raised through charity. The success of the 1927 flood relief effort earned Hoover the sobriquet the "Hero of the Flood" and carried him to the White House in the 1928 elections.

In the late spring and summer of 1930, a different, more insidious disaster unfolded over the Delta and surrounding regions of the South. In the last week of May, the rains stopped, and temperatures soared all through June, July, and August. Cotton plants withered in their rows, garden vegetables turned dry and brown, and mules scrounged for grass to feed on. Ponds and streams dried up, while the mighty Mississippi receded to the lowest levels ever recorded. Southern Arkansas was a scene of arid desolation: "Whirling dust boils up from gravel roadbeds, enveloping the trees and hollyhocks. Everything is the same monochromatic tan: people, trees, flowers and dogs."[21] As July turned into August, word reached Washington that much of the nation east of the Rockies was suffering one of the worst droughts in history, threatening not only the livelihood of millions of farmers but the nation's food supply. In the White House, President Hoover convened the governors of the ten hardest-hit states and the head of the Red Cross and outlined his drought relief program. Following his beliefs in self-help and voluntarism, each affected town, county, and state would form a relief committee, all of them guided by the National Drought Relief Committee. A Red Cross representative on each committee would help coordinate the work, direct relief supplies, and communicate any instructions from Washington. As in 1927, Hoover also encouraged regional banks to extend credit to farmers and negotiated with railroads to lower transportation rates for supplies into drought-stricken areas. These strategies had worked during the Great Flood; there was no reason they shouldn't succeed in 1930.

Unfortunately for farmers in the eight hardest-hit states, the much-vaunted drought relief plan did little to alleviate suffering. The present disaster was far different from the 1927 flood, covering a much broader area and affecting many more people. The Red Cross leadership was also far less enthusiastic about combating drought than flood. Although its charter called for the Red Cross to provide aid for all natural disasters, the leaders defined the drought as an economic hazard, lumping it among "strikes, business depressions, failure of crops and all other forms of unemployment and economic maladjustment which may cause widespread suffering."[22] Besides, they had strong reasons for dragging their heels on drought aid: hardship was so widespread that they were afraid that making an all-out effort to combat it would decimate their organization's finances.

Under pressure from Hoover, the Red Cross earmarked $5 million for drought relief but by the end of 1930 had spent only $460,000, mostly on seed distribution and far less on emergency food and clothing. Instead of leading the charge, it sought to shift the burden onto local communities. Their economies weakened by both drought and the larger business downturn, towns and cities in the drought area were in no shape to raise large amounts of money for relief. Between November 1930 and February 1931, more than five hundred banks across the region failed. Local business leaders also downplayed the effects of the drought, afraid that accepting relief would sap the work ethic and tar the region as a charity case. In the Delta, plantation owners denied that their sharecroppers were hungry. They had a long tradition of using food to control their poor black and white workers. Convinced that hungry workers would pick cotton more readily than those whose bellies were full of relief rations, bosses planned to pay their sharecroppers only half what they had received in years past for the harvest.

Hunger and privation continued across the drought area, and as the season turned colder, desperate farmers in the hard-hit states like Arkansas deluged the Red Cross with letters delineating their plight and pleading for aid. A woman in Magnolia, Arkansas, wrote that she and her children lacked both food and clothing and worried for their survival: "I am near at my row's end. I am asking you for help or advice some way."[23] A local Red Cross worker in western Arkansas wrote that most of the banks had failed and two hundred families needed immediate aid: "If you will investigate, you will find honest Americans here in Sevier County almost upon starvation."[24] Another visited forty-four sharecropper homes in the Delta and found only four men who were receiving wages. The families lived on flour, meal, lard, beans, and salt pork; none had fresh vegetables or dairy products; three families owned chickens, and one had a small pig.[25] On Christmas Day 1930, Albert Evans, the state Red Cross director, returned to the Delta expecting to find some sort of holiday cheer. Instead, he discovered that sharecroppers hadn't received any food from plantation owners, and only a handful had been granted Red Cross rations:

> A widow and seven children exemplified their plight. Their cupboard held a pint of flour and a few scraps of chicken bones, evidently the remains of their previous evening's meal. The only other food in the house consisted of twenty cans of fruit and vegetables the mother had put up during the summer. Their neighbors fared no better, living in cold cabins pasted with newspapers and eating remnants of lard and meal. One family of ten lived on a few pounds of rice, flour, beans, and lard, but all of the children were almost naked. Perhaps the most destitute he visited was a white family who had just eaten the last of their flour. Despite these conditions, Evans found no hysteria; instead, people just sat around their fires uncomplaining.[26]

Relief workers saw that pellagra and other malnutrition diseases were spreading. With winter now upon them, many more farm families would become ill, and some, particularly the old and very young, would surely die.

Nine days later, farmers' anger boiled over in the town of England, Arkansas, which was set in the middle of cotton fields on the Arkansas River's floodplain. A prime mover in the events of January 3, 1931, was a tenant farmer named Coney, who told his story to a writer for the *New Republic*:

> *We all got pretty low on food here, and some was a-starvin'. Mebbe I was a little better fixed than most, 'cause we still had some food left. But when a woman comes over to me a-cryin' and tells me her kids hain't et' nothin' fer two days, and grabs me and says, "Coney, what are we a-goin' to do?" then somethin' went up in my head. I just says, "Lady, you wait here. I'm a-goin' to get some food." Then I cranks up my truck you see settin' over yonder, and takes my wife and rolls over to Bell's place. Bell's the feller them Red Cross guys picks to run the relief, but he never give out nothin'. He always tell 'em he hain't got no blanks [relief applications] and they gotta wait. Well, I rolls over to Bell's place and finds a crowd of hungry men and Bell still a-sayin' that he hain't got no blanks. So I hollers out, "All you that hain't yaller, climb on my truck. We're a-goin' into England to get some grub." They all load onto her—forty-seven clum on, and let me tell you there warn't a one among 'em that had a gun of any sort.*[27]

In town, the hungry farmers went first to the police chief and the mayor to tell them that they had run out of food. Then they gathered in front of a grocery store while officials frantically called Albert Evans in the state Red Cross headquarters. The owner of another grocery store told his workers that if the crowd busted in, let them take the food but save the cash register. Meanwhile, the small group of protesters had attracted a larger crowd, apparently almost of all of them hungry farmers. Finally, an official arrived with blank forms, and by the end of the day the Red Cross had handed out two weeks' supply of food to five hundred families. Coney was pleased at the result:

> *Yes, sir, my gang stuck all right. I wouldn't a 'taken 'em if I hadn't a thought so. It wouldn't a' wanted but jest a little bit sass ter've had a showdown. But they doled out the feed and we all rolled back here without nobody gettin' hurt.*[28]

The following day, front-page headlines blared on newspapers across the country: "Arkansas Farmers Cry for Food, Riot." According to the Associated Press, at least five hundred farmers "stormed" England's business district demanding food, or else. Many were obviously armed, with pistols bulging from beneath their coats. When a local lawyer named George E. Morris attempted to calm them, they interrupted his speech with shouts of "We are not going to let our children starve!" and "We want food and we want it now!"[29] Morris told a reporter:

> *It was pathetic to hear these men and women crying for food, telling us their children actually were starving. . . . The crowd was really not wild, considering everything, but they were in earnest and it was not until I was able to tell them arrangements had been made for food that they would listen. They then quieted down and soon the merchants were doing everything they could to feed them.*[30]

Still, Morris worried about what would happen when the farmers ran out of their supplies of relief food: "The merchants of England either must move their goods or mount machine guns on their stores."[31]

News of what became known as the Arkansas "food riot" galvanized a debate already under way in Washington. After the com-
pletion of the harvest at the end of November, Cotton Belt leaders
suddenly decided that many of their farmers were in dire need of
help and might not survive the winter. In early December, Congressman James Benjamin Aswell of Louisiana proposed a bill giving
up to $60 million in animal feed, seed, fertilizer loans, and food to
stricken farmers. For President Hoover, the bill was anathema, a raid
on the Treasury that opened the door for the dreaded "dole" in the
form of food relief. Instead, he submitted a bill giving only $25 mil-
lion in loans and specifically forbidding food relief. In a House debate, Hoover supporter Congressman James Tilson called Aswell's
bill "revolutionary" and predicted: "The high principled and industrious among the distressed will insist on treating it as a loan and will
cripple themselves and their families in an attempt to repay it, and
the idle and shiftless will accept it as a gift, dismiss any attempt at
repayment, and live off the Federal Government as long as the opportunity exists."[32] What's more, federal relief would bypass the Red
Cross and thus "atrophy one of the noblest emotions of the human
heart—that of a generous response to a call for succor to distressed
peoples."[33] In the Senate, however, the Democrats were scathing in
their attacks on Hoover, accusing him of "playing politics with human misery." Senator Joseph Taylor Robinson of Arkansas ironically
summed up the debate: "It is all right to put a mule on the dole, but
terrible to put a man on one."[34] Meanwhile, the Red Cross continued
to drag its heels. Its chairman, John Barton Payne, told Congress:

> *In solving the many economic and social problems arising from*
> *the drought, it was considered essential that the Red Cross re-*
> *main in the background in so far as possible. The welfare of the*
> *individual drought sufferer could best be promoted by having*
> *him solve his own problem, if he could, through normal bank-*
> *ing and commercial channels. It was best that he secure other*

*employment if possible and work out his own recovery, relying*
*on the Red Cross only when his own efforts were unsuccessful.*[35]

Meanwhile, the events in England prompted big northern newspapers to send special correspondents down to Arkansas. They found Little Rock filled with bums and hoboes and politicians arguing about the dole. In smaller towns, banks were closed and stores were empty of customers despite big SALE signs in their windows. The only businesses that attracted a crowd were Red Cross offices, where farmers waited to sign up for relief. The need was growing, but it was clear that the Red Cross would require many millions more in order to adequately combat winter hunger.

Pushed by Hoover, on January 12, John Barton Payne announced that the Red Cross would mount a $10 million fundraising drive to meet the "greatly increased demands" of the previous ten days. Three days later, the president signed a compromise bill pledging $45 million for feed, seed, and fertilizer loans, but no food relief. Senators and congressmen from the drought area continued to push for federal food aid, pointing out that the Red Cross fund drive would raise only a fraction of the necessary money. Hoover and his conservative allies in Congress held firm in opposition, claiming that federal relief would destroy the Red Cross and be an "unwarranted" expansion of the federal government. Determined to squelch the opposition once and for all, on February 4, President Hoover delivered a national radio speech laying out his reasons for blocking federal money being used for "charitable purposes."

Hoover's address focused on the needs of both rural drought sufferers and the urban unemployed in the ongoing economic crisis. He began on a conciliatory note: "This is not an issue as to whether people shall go hungry or cold in the United States. It is solely a question of the best method by which hunger and cold shall be prevented." His opponents demanded to use federal dollars; Hoover wanted to preserve the "spirit of charity and mutual self-help through voluntary giving and the responsibility of local Government":

> *My own conviction is strongly that if we break down this sense of responsibility of individual generosity to individual and mutual self-help in this country in times of national difficulty, and if we start appropriations of this character, we have not only impaired something infinitely valuable in the life of the American people but have struck at the roots of government.*

As for urban unemployment, Hoover proposed a combination of federal public works programs along with charitable relief and help from local governments. If these policies did not work, he would then be open to changing course:

> *I am willing to pledge myself that if the time should ever come that the voluntary agencies of the country together with the local and state governments are unable to find resources with which to prevent hunger and suffering I will ask the aid of every resource of the Federal Government, because I would no more see starvation among our countrymen than would any Senator or Congressman.*

His opponents wanted him to begin these drastic measures immediately. However, Hoover was sure that he could avoid this "disastrous course," because he had "faith in the American people that such a day will not come."[36]

Down in the drought region, news that the Red Cross would soon begin to distribute food and clothing led almost half a million families to sign up at the local relief office. More than a third of them were in hard-hit rural Arkansas. Many had been living on a near starvation diet of salt pork, cornmeal, and turnips, or

"Hoover apples," the main harvest of the Red Cross seed distribution program back in the fall. One sharecropper remembered the desperation of that time:

> *We done without. I remember one time we got down to where we had nothin' for bread. But we had some nubbins of corn out in our barn. We took a bucket lid and nail, drove holes in it and went out there and got some of those nubbins and rubbed it across there to make meal out of so Mama could make corn bread.*[37]

Relief workers doled out a carefully measured "living diet" but not a "working diet," that is, enough to keep recipients from starving to death but not enough to give them energy to work. If lucky enough to receive a full monthly ration, a family of five would receive thirty-six pounds of flour, twenty-four pounds of split beans, twelve pounds of cracked rice, two pounds of coffee, twenty-four pounds of cornmeal, a half gallon of molasses, lard and bacon, and baking powder. Nutritionally speaking, this was only a slight improvement over the traditional "three m" diet, thanks to the addition of those beans, which were the cheapest available on the market:

> *Back in 1930 I remember the Red Cross giving us sacks of beans that had rocks in them. It was just like they had gone out there and piled up along a rocky place and loaded the rocks, which were the same color as those beans. You'd have to be real careful if Mama failed to catch the rocks when she was cooking them.*[38]

To help families make up the dietary deficiency, Red Cross representatives also handed out copies of a pamphlet called "The Family's Food at Low Cost," published by the USDA's Bureau of Home Economics. It suggested that children get milk at every meal; that potatoes, tomatoes, and green or yellow vegetables be served at least once a day; and that eggs, legumes, and lean meat be served two to four times a week. In the context of Arkansas, the most bankrupt state of the union in the blighted winter of 1930 to 1931, there was little chance that a farm family on relief could follow those recommendations. That was not a matter of Red Cross concern, according to national headquarters, because "Red Cross policy in disaster relief does not undertake to provide a more liberal standard of living than those existing in normal times."[39] When journalists grimly noted the rise of pellagra and other malnutrition diseases, the Red Cross sent its medical director, Dr. William DeKleine, to tour the area:

> *My recent visit through the drought areas of Arkansas, Louisiana, Mississippi, and Kentucky leads me to believe that the present shortage of food in these sections will not materially affect the general health of the people. . . . In all the homes and schools I visited I did not find any evidence of malnutrition more than exists in normal times. . . . I can, therefore, see no particular reason for alarm over health problems that may develop because of the present shortage of food, unless it is recognized that these problems have existed for a long time. . . . This does not mean that no attempt should be made to promote better food habits, but rather that under the circumstances the most important thing to do is to provide food for the hungry and actually prevent starvation. . . . Hungry families want food, and they want the kind they know and like the best. Folks who are accustomed to using flour, meal, salt meat, molasses, lard, rice, beans, and coffee, want these now, and the relief agencies must furnish these staples. The habits of a people cannot be changed overnight.[40]*

The Red Cross also allowed local chapters wide leeway in setting rules about food relief. In Arkansas cotton country, local leaders remembered the aftermath of the 1927 flood, when many sharecroppers had been "allowed to loaf and eat."[41] One planter said: "Lord I hate to see my niggers . . . put on any kind of free dole. It's their salvation to have to work for what they get."[42] Many Delta Red Cross chapters required black sharecroppers, but not whites, to work on street repairs or in the fields before they could receive rations. This was in violation of Red Cross rules, which specified that relief could be distributed only on the basis of need, with no strings attached. Blacks who protested were beaten or simply denied food.

In some areas, relief supplies were distributed by the planters themselves, who often skimped on amounts to ensure a hungry and therefore eager workforce. After complaints from local black leaders and the NAACP, the Red Cross investigated and confirmed the accounts. One country Red Cross chairman told the national office: "If people get it into their heads that when they have made a little cotton crop and tried to make a corn crop and failed and then expected charity to feed them for five months, then the Red Cross had defeated the very thing that it should have promoted, self-reliance and initiative."[43] Rather than punish the local chapters, Red Cross leaders simply shook their heads and, at the end of March, wound down the distribution of food relief. Secretary of Agriculture Arthur Hyde toured the region and returned to report that he saw no signs of human suffering:

> *Everywhere people were putting in gardens and preparing the ground for crops. The drought had been broken by rains, and if it would only stay broken by receiving the normal precipitation from now on all would be well.*

Indeed, the only complaint of any kind he had encountered was from an old man by the roadside who said the Red Cross had "fed them too well."[44]

Thanks to the richness of their land, the citizens of Arkansas and other Delta regions managed a partial recovery from the linked effects of drought and economic slowdown. At least they were able to grow enough food to feed their families, after a fashion. Other parts of the South were less lucky. Although Arkansas was hardest hit by the drought, a belt of devastation also stretched north and east into Missouri, Tennessee, Kentucky, West Virginia, and Virginia. Much of this region was Southern Appalachia, home to thousands of small subsistence farms, many miles from the nearest road. In the mountains of southeastern Kentucky, there were only a few towns, usually the county seats, of a few hundred people each:

> All the rest of the mountaineers lived in lonely cabins and shacks scattered along the rivers and up the creeks and branches that made deep cut into the hills. Those narrow canyons were their homes. The steep slopes and ridges above them, covered with fine forests of poplar, black walnut, oak and beech, made free feeding grounds for their hogs. . . . On small strips of rocky soil on the slopes and down in the creek bottoms, they raised corn for their huge families and for the winter feeding of their cows and sheep, if they had them, ducks, geese and chickens, mules and hogs. And in autumn came the "foddering"—whole families working early and late to get in the corn before the rains. . . . For most of the people in the hills, corn pone and potatoes and pork was their food, three times a day, year in and year out.[45]

This precarious mode of life persisted across the mountains from Kentucky all the way to Virginia's Blue Ridge Mountains, where people lived much as the first settlers had 150 years earlier. They survived by hunting, fishing, logging, and planting a few small fields. In winter they ate cornmeal, cabbage, dried apples, and salt pork, with an occasional squirrel or rabbit; in summer their diet was supplemented by fresh greens and other vegetables, fish, beans, and milk.[46] Few of the children attended school or even knew the name of the president.

When the 1930 drought hit the mountains of Appalachia, the heat and lack of rain blackened cornfields and dried up wells and springs. Farm animals had to be slaughtered because there was no forage for them. Men picked up their rifles and went into the woods, decimating the local population of deer, squirrel, rabbit, and birds. After the corn crop failed, people had no surplus to last them through the winter. By January, the situation was so bad that a desperate Kentucky Red Cross worker wrote:

> *We have done our best for everybody. We have filled up the poor farm. We have carted our children to orphanages for the sake of feeding them. There is no more room. Our people in the country are starving and freezing.*[47]

The national Red Cross granted the hungry people a bare-bones $1.50 to $2.50 a month food ration. Down in the county seats, many local chapter leaders thought even that was too much for the hill folk, whom they saw as more or less subhuman, mostly criminals and moonshiners. After a tour of Kentucky, Dr. William DeKleine of the Red Cross wrote: "There is a feeling among the better farmers in Boyd County that the drought is providential; that God intended the dumb ones should be wiped out; and that it is a mistake to feed them."[48] God, it seems, had a different idea. In April 1931, the rains resumed, and hill folk once again began hoeing their fields and planting their gardens (often with Red Cross seed).

Subsistence farmers made up only a portion of Appalachia's population. Large tracts of eastern Kentucky and West Virginia sat on a vast deposit of relatively clean-burning bituminous coal. Coalfields were discovered there in 1750, but isolation and lack of a railroad precluded commercial mining (another monoculture, but this time of fossilized plant matter) until the late nineteenth century. Coal prices soared during World War I, driving up wages and luring men from their hill farms to jobs in the mines. However, the boom ended when European coalfields resumed production, and by 1927 wages and hours began to slide downward. To make up for the loss of profits, mine operators were as creative as cotton plantation owners in finding new ways to squeeze every last dollar out of their workers. Miners and their families lived in company-owned houses as drafty and poorly built as sharecroppers' shacks down in the Delta. They got their water from local springs and streams, often typhoid-ridden and gritty with coal dust. The miners were paid not in cash but in company "scrip" from which owners deducted the worker's rent, coal for heating his house, blasting powder for use in the mines, and "expenses" that included substandard medical care and contributions to a burial fund. With what was left, the miner's wife could go to the company store to buy food, at prices that were easily double those found in the closest town.

The family diet was based on beans, cornbread, salt pork, and "bulldog gravy" made from flour, water, and grease. Fresh milk was nearly unobtainable, and in any case miners had no money to pay local farmers. If they could find a little plot of land, they might be able to scratch out a few vegetables during the summertime (if there was rain). Children rarely attended school and were often sickly. Many older miners suffered from black lung disease, and almost all owed debts to the company store that they could never repay.

Life in Appalachia's coalfields had long been marked by labor unrest, which frequently turned into outright violence. One of the few relief valves for this tension was the mines' proximity to the hills; when conditions got too bad, many miners would just return to their mountain farms. However, in the drought-wracked winter of 1930 to 1931, the farms were not producing. Then, in February 1931, mine operators in Harlan County, Kentucky, squeezed by the economic depression, announced a 10 percent wage cut for all workers. The United Mine Workers Union quickly called a mass meeting to exhort miners to unionize in order to block wage cuts and improve working conditions. The next day, mine operators began firing any workers who attended and evicting them and their families from company housing. These actions sparked a decade-long conflict marked by violence, strikes, legal battles, and widespread deprivation that spread across the coalfields of Appalachia. Harlan County, which already bristled with guns, was particularly bloody, with dozens of men dying on both sides of the battle. Caught in between were the striking miners' wives and children, who huddled in makeshift camps while the men fought for better wages. For food, they had little more than beans, salt pork, and cornbread; with no milk, many infants and small children died of malnutrition. Many had been helped into the world by Molly Jackson, a nurse and union worker's wife who in the fall of 1931 wrote a song called "Kentucky Miner's Wife (Ragged Hungry Blues)":

> *I'm sad and weary; I've got the hungry ragged blues;*
> *I'm sad and weary; I've got the hungry ragged blues;*
> *Not a penny in my pocket to buy the thing I need to use.*
> *I woke up this morning with the worst blues I ever had in my life;*
> *I woke up this morning with the worst blues I ever had in my life;*
> *Not a bite to cook for breakfast, a poor coal miner's wife . . .*

> *. . . This mining town I live in is a sad and lonely place,*
> *This mining town I live in is a sad and lonely place,*
> *Where pity and starvation are pictured on every face.*

> *Ragged and hungry, no slippers on our feet,*
> *Ragged and hungry, no slippers on our feet,*
> *We're bumming around from place to place to get a little bite to eat.*

*All a-going round from place to place bumming for a little food to eat.*
*Listen, my friends and comrades, please take a friend's advice,*
*Don't put out no more of your labor, till you get a living price.*

*Some coal operators might tell you the hungry blues are not bad;*
*Some coal operators might tell you the hungry blues are not bad;*
*They are the worst blues this poor woman ever had.*[49]

In most places in Appalachia, there existed no state-run relief organizations and only a bare-bones local relief apparatus, usually with enough funds to run the county poorhouse and support a few of the "aged, blind, and chronically sick." Hungry workers turned first to the UMW, but the union quickly backed off its commitment to the Harlan strike. The Harlan County Red Cross chapter had recently been given $3,000 by the national office. However, the coal companies controlled its leadership, which reiterated organization policy about providing food relief in natural disasters but not industrial downturns. Exceptions were made only for those few miners who had managed to find a plot of land for growing vegetables—Red Cross rules said they could be aided as farmers. As for striking miners in Harlan County, they were bluntly told: "You want relief? Go back to work."

In other parts of coal country, mine workers faced slowly decreasing work hours and the unrelenting economics of the company store. In West Virginia, their plight became so dire that Brant Scott, a state mine union leader, traveled to Washington to plead for aid, telling senators that a third of the state's 112,000 miners were unemployed and another third worked only one or two days a week. In mine settlements, many children ran around half naked and shoeless and suffered from rickets. In the Kanawha region, home to about 25,000 miners, Scott estimated that 8,000 workers were "hungry and destitute." He added: "Their diet is potatoes, bread, beans, oleomargarine, but not meat, except sow-belly two or three times a week. The company won't let the miners keep cows or pigs and the children almost never have fresh milk. Only a few get even canned milk."[50] Scott had received nothing from state Red Cross officials: "They would not give any reason except that they were not sending relief to the rural regions. . . . I visited them three times. They know the conditions, but still they won't be giving them."[51] The senators immediately set up a meeting for Scott at Red Cross headquarters to state his case. President Hoover also wrote to John Barton Payne asking him to help the miners: "There is no doubt some real suffering and it is likely to be formulated as a charge that the Red Cross is not taking care of the whole of the people in that area."[52] Once again, Payne refused, fearing that this would open the door to Red Cross responsibility for much wider unemployment relief. However, he did not want to sound totally heartless: "We have offered seed for planting wherever the miners can find land on which to plant."[53]

John Barton Payne had repeatedly blocked the administration's aid requests, causing severe political damage to the president. Somehow, Hoover's affection for the organization never wavered. He was guest of honor at the Red Cross's fiftieth anniversary dinner, where he praised Payne for "his steadfastness in holding the organization to its national ideal as a non-governmental agency for the free expression of the private generosity and humanity of the people." Meanwhile, the situation in the Appalachian coal-fields continued to deteriorate as strikes and hunger spread.

Pushed by dire news reports, Hoover aides contacted the American Friends Service Committee, a Quaker relief organization, to see if it could help the miners. The Friends recognized that "the condition in the bituminous coal field represents a collapse of civilization at a critical point."[54] They agreed to feed hungry children in the coal areas, but only if they could also help train laid-off miners and their wives in other types of work. Hoover promised them $200,000, to be provided by the Red Cross. The

Friends waited for two months, and finally Payne responded: "For the Red Cross to provide funds in the face of need in several states would, I fear, involve serious criticism—more than if nothing was done."[55] Somehow, Hoover found $225,000 in an idle account belonging to a World War I European relief organization and immediately sent it to the Friends. They set up stations in Kentucky, West Virginia, Pennsylvania, Illinois, Maryland, and Tennessee to give milk and "one substantial meal" to up to forty thousand children a day. Pregnant and nursing mothers were also fed; Quaker volunteers taught miners' wives how to sew and their idle husbands how to craft furniture. This program allowed Hoover to give relief without using federal funds, the Red Cross to protect its narrowly defined mission, and mine owners and local politicians to preserve their power. Nevertheless, Quaker relief fed only a small segment, albeit the most vulnerable one, of the hundreds of thousands of hungry and malnourished people across Appalachia.

# Chapter 5

————◦◦◦————

OUR PURITAN ANCESTORS took it as an article of faith that the idle were unworthy of charity, a sentiment famously captured by the Calvinist preacher Cotton Mather: "For those who indulge themselves in idleness, the express command of God unto us is, that we should let them starve."[1] Long after Mather departed this world, his spirit lived on, embodied in the nation's poor laws. Statutes that outlined government's responsibility to the destitute, the poor laws combined guarded concern for needy Americans with suspicions that they were complicit in their own misfortune. Under the poor laws, the chronically jobless were removed from society and dispatched to county poorhouses, catchall institutions that were also home to the old, infirm, and mentally ill. Those who could ordinarily shift for themselves but were temporarily jobless applied to public officials, men with no special welfare training, for what was known as outdoor or home relief, assistance generally given in the form of food and coal. To discourage idlers, the welfare experience was made as unpleasant as possible. Before applying for help, the poor were made to wait until utterly penniless, and then declare it publicly. When granting relief, officers followed the old rule of thumb that families living "on the town" must never reach the comfort level of the poorest independent family. The weekly food allowance was a meager four dollars a week—and less in some areas—regardless of how many people it was supposed to feed. Finally, it was customary to give food and coal on alternate weeks, providing minimal nourishment and warmth, but never both at the same time.

By custom and by law, public relief in the United States had always been a local concern, the responsibility of towns, cities, and counties. By the summer of 1931, however, in communities across the United States the money raised for the jobless had evaporated, while the numbers of people applying for it continued to climb. Still, Hoover remained confident that between private charity and local government, America would find its way out of the job crisis. An announcement from the White House in August made it official: the president was against a federal dole and was not about to support one. In Albany, Governor Franklin Delano Roosevelt took the news as his cue, and on August 29, 1931, he proposed the creation of the Temporary Emergency Relief Administration. This state program for helping the unemployed drastically expanded government's responsibility to care for its people. In times of crisis, Roosevelt argued, government was obliged to help the victims of adverse circumstance, providing them with shelter, clothing, and food, "not as a matter of charity, but as a matter of social duty." When TERA was passed into law that September, for the first time in the country's history a state government assumed the job of feeding the hungry.

In the months of deliberation leading up to TERA, social workers became Roosevelt's eyes and ears. The governor consulted with social worker Homer Folks, the author of two major reports on living conditions around the state, who impressed on Roosevelt the necessity of taking action. Formulating his plans for emergency relief, Roosevelt looked to social workers for guidance, and when it was time to staff his administration he chose social worker Harry Hopkins for the job of director. Forty-two years old at the time, Hopkins was a gangly chain smoker and drinker of black coffee, habits that accentuated his own natural stores of nervous energy. From his first job with a settlement house, he had channeled that energy into his career, climbing, job by job, from field worker to director of the New York Tuberculosis Association. Directing TERA would require the sum of his professional experiences.

TERA was conceived of as a kind of task force. The original staff of fifty, many of them social workers and more than half volunteers, set up their command center in Manhattan on East Twenty-Eighth Street, with the idea that it would operate from November to June. Though the center's run was brief, organizers were impressed by the magnitude of their endeavor. In the minds of its creators, TERA marked the arrival of a welfare system that was rational and efficient but also compassionate. Its centerpiece

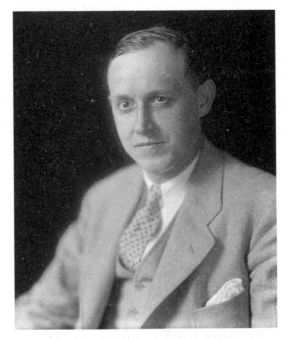

*Harry Hopkins, also known as the "minister of relief."* (Harris & Ewing Collection, Library of Congress, LC-DIG-hec-21642)

was a public works program through which jobless men and women could earn an honest wage—which was always preferable to handouts—but the administration's first objective was preventing starvation.

Food relief under TERA was one front in the welfare revolution, its manifesto a thirty-page manual issued by the new administration and distributed to officials across the state. Where public welfare traditionally observed a one-size-fits-all policy, food relief under TERA was rationalized, each distribution calculated to feed households of different size and composition. Under the old welfare regime, humiliation was brandished like a stick. TERA aspired to more considerate methods. The application process began with an interview at the local welfare office, conducted behind closed doors to preserve privacy. Since the person doing the interviewing was a member of the old public welfare regime, he was supervised by a TERA social worker, thus ensuring a policy of "kindly consideration."[2] To avoid public lines and similar spectacles, qualified households received weekly grocery orders, which, like coupons, could be discreetly traded in for food at the local market. Finally, in distinction to the premeditated stinginess of the past, food relief under the new administration had to be *adequate*. In early TERA planning sessions, the question was raised of whether adequate relief, defined by TERA as sufficient to "prevent physical suffering" and "maintain a minimal living standard," would remove the incentive to work. The answer was yes, but only if the Depression dragged on for years, which was inconceivable.

The Depression's many emergency diets, including the one issued by TERA, belong to a history of nutritional guidance for the poor that began with Atwater at the turn of the century. To help ensure a productive workforce, in 1894 Atwater established America's first dietary standards, nutritional recommendations directed at the nation's wage earners that were based on levels of physical exertion. So, for example, a watchman required more nutrients than a clerk but fewer than a carpenter, each man consuming only the food required to perform his daily labors. Using the man of the family as his reference point, Atwater then calculated the food needs of women and children, a bizarrely illogical formula. (Should the family of a tailor receive half as much nourishment as that of a street paver?) Over the next two decades, the standards were widely adopted by hospitals, schools, and other institutions. They were also embraced by private charities, which used them as a basis for food relief, bringing Atwater into the home.

In 1917, the year America entered World War I, the nation received some unsettling health news. According to the draft bureau, of the millions of men called to serve—young men in their supposed prime—more than a third were physically unfit for combat, many with conditions caused by poor diet like rickets and bad teeth. The start of food conservation later that year unleashed a new round of nutritional worries. The sharp rise in food prices caused by conservation had set off a corresponding increase in childhood malnutrition. The hardest hit were poor families living in cities like New York, where Board of Health inspectors reported that one-eighth of the city's schoolchildren were underfed.[3] As food authorities shifted their attention from the worker to the child, health agencies opened free nutrition clinics, mounted food exhibitions, and issued instructional leaflets. Newspapers printed special children's menus and recipes that were both conservation-minded and nutritious, all part of a sweeping educational campaign directed at American homemakers.

Lucy Gillett was a New York nutritionist who worked for one of the city's oldest and largest charities, the Association for Improving the Condition of the Poor. In 1917, just as childhood malnutrition was grabbing newspaper headlines, Gillett was finishing her own study on the subject. Among her conclusions was the fact that children fed on Atwater's standards were suffering the consequences, kept alive in a state of semi-starvation. In place of Atwater's fractions, Gillett proposed that nutritionists treat each family member on his or her own merits, according to that person's age, size, and level of activity.[4] Gillett's 1918 *Food Primer for the Home*, one of the many nutrition manuals published during the war, stressed the importance of ample feeding, assuring mothers that there was little danger of eating too much of a balanced diet. Good nutrition, moreover, was within the grasp of rich and poor alike, as easy to achieve as following these basic guidelines:

> *Spend no more for meat than for milk . . .*
> *Spend as much or more for vegetables and fruit as for meat . . .*
> *Eat freely of cereals and bread to satisfy the appetite . . .*[5]

Though nutritionists and welfare workers shared overlapping concerns, Gillett was an early example of someone who combined them in one job. (On her retirement in 1944 she was described as "the first nutritionist to work in the welfare field.") At the intersection of these two emerging professions, she could appreciate the importance of balancing economy on the one hand with the nutritional requirements for good health on the other. Her compromise was an "adequate minimum food allowance," a weekly grocery order below which health was at risk. Gillett worked out a method for arriving at that dollar amount—which of course would vary from family to family and region to region—allowing charities to dispense food dollars with scientific precision and efficiency.

While the country tended to nutrition problems at home, the more pressing food crisis was unfolding thousands of miles away in war-torn Europe. Under Herbert Hoover's leadership, the United States Food Administration responded with a relief program ambitious enough to feed a continent. Americans were encouraged to curtail their consumption of beef, pork, wheat, butter, and sugar, while their government fed Allied troops and millions of refugees in Europe. In the first years of the Great Depression, with the war still alive in people's memories, the nation experienced a sense of déjà vu. Another food emergency was at hand, only this time the hungry masses were here on American soil.

In a replay of 1917, nutritionists and other food authorities jumped in with advice. Newspapers began to print suggestions for budget menus recommending the temporary suspension of America's normal eating habits. Most dramatically, families accustomed to two meat meals a day would have to cut back to only three or four a *week*, presenting a creative challenge to the home cook. Satisfying the family with a standing rib roast was easy, but how would the home cook do the same with lima beans? To this question, the authorities had a ready answer: "The fact that a really good cook can serve better meals on a small budget than a poor cook can serve on the fat of the land suggests that the fault may be not in the food material itself but in the manner in which the food is prepared and served, and therein lays a tale!"[6] So the gauntlet was thrown.

Columnists who wrote for the women's pages exhorted home cooks to raise the level of their game and master new skills. To imbue those beans with savor, women would learn to cook them with a piece of beef fat saved from the night before. Soup making, which required only bones, was an essential skill, and for those occasions when meat was available, homemakers would have to brush up on braising and stewing, cooking methods best suited to the cheapest parts of the animal. But more enticing than either soups or stews was cooking *en casserole*. A food column favorite, casserole cookery was well suited to inexpensive ingredients, it was easy to serve and to clean up after, and, like all one-pot meals, a casserole saved on fuel costs. Best of all was its endless flexibility, inviting women to experiment with whatever was on hand. A story on casserole cooking in the *New York Herald Tribune* hinted at the possibilities:

> *lima beans, onions, green peppers and tomatoes en casserole; Spanish rice; stuffed eggplant; vegetable loaf or vegetable pies; baked peas and bacon; rice baked with cheese and tomatoes; corned beef hash au gratin; baked liver with vegetables and macaroni; scalloped salmon, stuffed onions and stuffed peppers; tomatoes and lima beans en casserole; scalloped cauliflower; sweet potatoes and apples; tuna fish pie; stuffed beef heart; baked eggs au gratin; casserole of cheese and vegetables; Swiss steak with browned potatoes; cheese fondue; beef pie with pastry crust; lamb cutlets en casserole; shrimp creole; liver with spaghetti, baked dried fruit; baked meatballs with tomato sauce; baked beans with corn; baked onion soup.[7]*

Finally, the casserole dish was a place to hide foods people did not especially like. One of them was liver, another beans—two of the more common casserole ingredients. And if the family groaned at the sight of leftovers, casseroles allowed "budgeteers" to bury yesterday's dinner, now minced and coated in white sauce, under a veil of bread crumbs.

Casseroles were one of the Depression's many "mystery foods," inventions of necessity, which the cooking columns presented as feats of ingenuity. Hence the following snippet of imagined dinnertime conversation from Mary Meade, food columnist at the *Chicago Daily Tribune*:

> *"What is it?" demands father.*
> *"Guess!" challenges mother.*

*"Hash!" ventures Billy.*

*"Pie!" gurgles Mary.*

*But whatever the answer, it's bound to be an epic if mother is up to the minute on the art of turning homely foods into culinary triumphs.*[8]

Along the same mysterious lines but more so, just about any food could be ground up, mixed with bread crumbs and egg, then shaped into a loaf and baked until firm. Women's pages were flooded with loaf recipes that used beans, liver, and nuts, cheap and generally unloved forms of protein, as stand-ins for beef, pork, and chicken. It was clearly a budget food, but in the interest of public morale, Meade found reasons to sing its praises. All this new economizing, she wrote, had opened "a grand and glorious field for adventure in creating new tantalizing dishes in which the old faithfuls can take on new charms." It would be hard to describe the need for food budgeting in a sunnier light. The following is her recipe for pea roast:

1 egg well beaten

1 tablespoon sugar

¼ cup melted butter

½ cup pea pulp (canned or dried)

¼ cup finely chopped peanuts

¾ cup whole milk

¾ cup stale bread crumbs

salt and pepper to taste

Blend the melted butter with the sugar and eggs. Mix together the pea pulp, peanuts, seasonings, bread crumbs, and milk and combine with the first mixture. Turn into a greased pan and bake in a moderate oven (350 degrees F.) 25 minutes. Serve with tomato sauce or chopped pickle. This interesting entrée comes to you for the pleasant sum of approximately 17 cents and serves four generously.[9]

———————

Whatever invention took place in the kitchen was dependent on the women's shopping acumen. Articles on smart marketing implored homemakers to think of themselves as businesswomen and keep grocery accounts, a good way to identify wasteful spending patterns and root them out. But the key to staying on budget was planning menus in advance, week by week, with no spur-of-the-moment purchases or concessions to gastronomic whim. By the fall of 1930, the New York newspapers had begun to print these budget menus, showing homemakers that it was possible, for example, to feed the family on twelve dollars a week. New budgets appeared every few weeks, each one lower than the one preceding it, demanding greater and greater marketing discipline.

Business girls living on their own had to exercise similar restraint at the neighborhood cafeteria, where so many of their meals were taken. In the winter of 1931, the YWCA put together a meal plan for the "dollar-a-day girl" that would provide her with 2,000 calories daily, the lowest possible number "consistent with good health and spirits." The following is a sample menu published in the New York newspapers based on local cafeteria offerings:

BREAKFAST
*Baked Apple with Cream*
*Two Slices Toast with Butter*
*Coffee Cream Sugar*

### Lunch

*Cream Soup*
*Peanut and Cheese Salad, or*
*Toasted Cheese Sandwich*
*Banana*

### Dinner

*Potatoes, Gravy*
*Cole Slaw, Mayonnaise*
*Custard or Pudding, Milk*[10]

More restrained still, for those on microscopic budgets, nutritionists designed fifty-cent-a-day menus in which "flavor satisfaction" was taken out of the equation. Intended mainly for students, the fifty-cent meal plan, though spare, had "everything essential for health and strength." Taking into account the different dietary needs of men and women, nutritionists offered a version for each gender:

### Breakfast in Room

#### MAN.

| | |
|---|---|
| *1 pt. milk* . . . . . . . . . . . . . . . . . . . . . | 0.05 |
| *¼ loaf whole wheat bread, sliced* . . . . . . . . . | 0.02 |
| *1 banana (possibly two)* . . . . . . . . . . . . . | <u>0.03</u> |
| | 0.10 |

#### WOMAN.

| | |
|---|---|
| *1 pt. milk* . . . . . . . . . . . . . . . . . . . . . | 0.05 |
| *1 shredded wheat biscuit* . . . . . . . . . . . . | 0.01 |
| *1 orange* . . . . . . . . . . . . . . . . . . . . . | 0.03 |
| *1 tsp. sugar* . . . . . . . . . . . . . . . . . . . | <u>0.003</u> |
| | 0.093 |

## LUNCH IN CAFETERIA

### MAN.

*Choose:*
*Milk in preference to coffee*
*Cream soup, not thin*
*Vegetables or salad always*
*Always take butter*

### WOMAN.

*(Same as Man's)* . . . . . . . . . . . . . . . . . . .  0.25

## SUPPER IN ROOM

### MAN.

*1 pt. milk (rest of the day's milk).* . . . . . . . . . .  0.05
*¼ lb. graham crackers.* . . . . . . . . . . . . . .  0.05
*1 pkg. raisins* . . . . . . . . . . . . . . . . . . .  <u>0.05</u>
                                                        0.15

### WOMAN.

*1 pt. milk, flavored with chocolate syrup.* . . . . . .  0.05
*(can be bought at 5-and-ten-cent*
*store for 10 cents)* . . . . . . . . . . . . . . . . .  0.01
*¼ loaf white bread* . . . . . . . . . . . . . . . . .  0.02
*1 banana (possibly two).* . . . . . . . . . . . . . .  <u>0.03</u>
                                                        0.11[11]

Food authorities understood that such spartan offerings delivered minimal eating pleasure but were confident that students would adjust to them quickly and in fact would come to feel better on them than on more expensive fare.

———•◦•———

UNDER NORMAL CIRCUMSTANCES, a homemaker could rely on taste and habit when preparing meals, and chances are the family would be relatively well nourished. Under economic pressure, however, that same woman faced less promising odds. A deeper understanding of food science was one way to improve those odds. "Families who are not familiar with food values," the experts warned, "are practicing a deadly sort of economy."[12] The grocery bill must be trimmed, but intelligently, accomplished with a firm command of basic nutrition.

Starting in 1931, a cascade of nutrition pamphlets, leaflets, and booklets began raining down on the American reading public. Available through schools, health departments, charities, and even the American Legion, they advised people to satisfy what nutritionists called the "hidden hunger." Here, again, ordinary men and women would have to find within themselves the self-discipline of an ascetic, ignoring the pangs in their bellies in deference to the body's undetected need for minerals and vitamins. After all, hunger pain was temporary, and so was hunger-induced weakness. A shortage of essential nutrients, on the other hand, opened the door to lasting injury, problematic for anyone but disastrous for children "who only grow but once." Many of these pamphlets came straight from the USDA's Bureau of Home Economics, the official government voice on all matters culinary. More were issued by private charities, but all relied on the rule of thumb first devised by Lucy Gillett's teacher and mentor, Henry Sherman, professor of chemistry at Columbia University, where Gillett had studied. According to Sherman, the food budget ideally should be divided into fifths, one for fruits and vegetables, one for milk, one for meat, one for cereals, and the last for fats.

In 1931, scrambling to put a staff together, Harry Hopkins naturally turned to people he knew from the social work community. Among them was Gillett, perhaps the one person in America best qualified to design the TERA diet. In its first month, TERA fed more than 38,000 New York families, but that number would rise, reaching a peak of 435,000 in 1935. The TERA diet, which gave first priority to the needs of children, followed the one-fifths formula, concentrating on foods high in calcium and vitamins A, B, and C. Accordingly, potatoes, cabbage, carrots, canned tomatoes, dried beans, and dried fruit, all vitamin-packed and cheap, made up the top tier in the TERA food hierarchy. At the pinnacle, however, milk was revered as the one food that contained all four of the protective nutrients and the only food for which there was no substitute. An elixir of health, milk was indispensable to children, for whom TERA allotted a quart a day, but was mandatory for adults as well, who could get by with only a pint.

The Depression's many emergency diets, including the one issued by TERA, were founded on repetition, mealtimes restricted to a select group of bargain foods. The inevitable result was boredom, a fact of life accepted by food scientists who warned against the enticements of a variety. "Let no one be misled by the extravagant phrase 'deadly monotony,'" was Professor Sherman's advice. "No deaths are ever caused by monotony of diet, if the diet, however simple and cheap, provides the actual necessary nutrients."[13] At least this was the view from on high. Closer to ground level, where real women faced the daily challenge of feeding the family, monotony was something to rally against. For homemakers daunted by the task of cooking with the same few ingredients week in and week out, inspiration was provided by a team of home economists at Cornell University.

Formed in 1908, the Cornell Department of Home Economics was under the dual command of Martha Van Rensselaer and Flora Rose, who not only worked together but lived together as lifelong companions. Sometimes referred to as "Miss Van Rose," both women belonged to the world of reformers and activists that included Eleanor Roosevelt. In fact, Rose and Roosevelt had met in the early 1920s through the League of Women Voters, that first encounter the start of an enduring friendship. The Van Roses were frequent houseguests at the Roosevelt estate in Hyde Park, and the Roosevelts made yearly pilgrimages to Cornell to speak at its Farm and Home Week. With the start of state-sponsored food relief in 1931, Rose and Van Rensselaer collaborated with TERA, creating relief menus that used only TERA-sanctioned foods, combined and recombined to give the illusion of variety. So, from her eighteen-pound ration of potatoes, a woman might prepare potato and onion soup one day, followed by potato omelet, potato hot pot, or scalloped potatoes baked in tomato sauce. The same tomato sauce was poured over deviled eggs, while whole onions were baked in it and eaten for lunch. Tomatoes were also scalloped on their own, the liquid from the can saved and served to the children at breakfast in place of orange juice.

The typical TERA family, consisting of husband, wife, and three or four children, received twenty-eight quarts of milk each week, some for the children to drink, the rest intended for use in cooking. With so much of it on hand, milk made regular appearances in the Cornell recipes, poured into chowders and puddings, baked into breads, and stirred into white sauce, one of the true workhorses of the American kitchen. A banner food of the domestic science movement, white sauce rose to culinary stardom at the tail end of the nineteenth century. The many stacks of cookbooks produced by home economists—Fannie Farmer's among them— all contained white sauce recipes, and every cooking school curriculum devoted a lesson to it. While the standard white sauce was made from two tablespoons of flour, two tablespoons of butter, and one cup of milk, it could be thinned or thickened according to use. Concealing otherwise naked foods under an ivory cloak, it was poured over vegetables, cold meats, seafood, eggs, and macaroni, elevating ordinary ingredients and tempering flavors that were too pronounced on their own. It was the "cream" in creamed chicken, creamed cod, creamed sweetbreads, and creamed tongue on toast. More discreetly, white sauce thickened soups, enriched

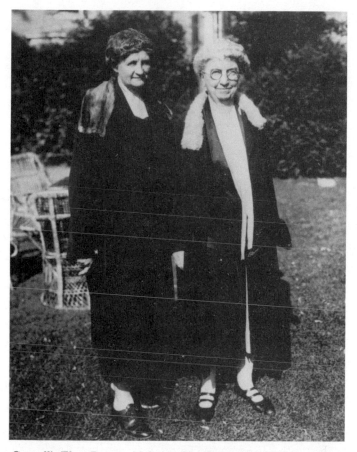

*Cornell's Flora Rose and Martha Van Rensselaer while visiting the Roosevelts in Hyde Park.* (Cornell University, Carl A. Kroch Library, Division of Rare and Manuscript Collections)

purees, was the binding agent in croquettes and the liquid component of anything "scalloped."

During the Depression, home economists like Flora Rose turned to white sauce as a medium for pumping nutrients into the American diet. Devising ways to use it, Rose had an immense oeuvre of recipes to choose from. Creamed carrots was an old standard. In this recipe, carrots, white sauce, and pasta, an inexpensive source of energy, are combined into an odd but nourishing casserole:

---

## Creamed Spaghetti with Carrots

1½ cups broken spaghetti

3 tablespoons margarine

3 tablespoons flour

½ teaspoon salt

⅛ teaspoon pepper

3 cups fresh or diluted evaporated milk

1½ cups cooked carrots

Clean and scrape carrots, cut in long, narrow slices and cook until tender in a small amount of boiling salted water. Cook the spaghetti until tender (about 25 minutes) in 3 quarts of boiled water to which has been added 1½ tablespoons of salt. Drain. Melt fat, add flour and seasonings and blend thoroughly. Pour on the milk and stir until thick and smooth. Cook for 5 minutes longer. Put one-half the spaghetti in a baking dish, cover with ½ carrots, then add ½ the sauce. Repeat, using the remaining ingredients. Bake in a moderate oven for 15 to 20 minutes.[14]

---

AS IT TURNED out, plans for temporary relief in New York were prematurely optimistic. Intended to run through the spring of 1932, by March of that year it was clear that TERA would have to be extended. But where the economic news was glum, the mood among TERA directors was congratulatory. In a progress report to the governor, Harry Hopkins called TERA "one of the greatest social experiments ever undertaken." Many doles had been tried before, he continued, but this was the first to sustain a great commonwealth "without a tinge of beggary," feeding a hungry public while sparing it humiliation.[15] This official view, however, was at odds with the experiences of those New Yorkers on the TERA relief rolls.

For a family to qualify for TERA, all of its assets had to be exhausted, a slow process of attrition that stopped only when there was nothing left to sell and no one left to borrow from. To ascertain that applicants were truly destitute, officials subjected them to a round of interviews. Candor was not assumed. Rather, all claims were verified through interviews with relatives and former employers, which was not only embarrassing but could hurt a man's chances for employment in the future.[16] More demeaning, however, were the home visits by TERA investigators to make sure the family's situation was sufficiently desperate. Investigators came once a month, unannounced, anxious to catch welfare abusers. Any sign that the family's finances had improved—a suspiciously new-looking dress or fresh set of window curtains—was grounds for cross-examination. If the man of the house was not at home—a suggestion that he might be out earning money—investigators asked for his whereabouts, collecting names and addresses for later verification. Finally, though instructed otherwise, investigators were known to reprimand women for becoming pregnant while on relief, the ultimate intrusion.[17] Families lived in dread of these monthly visits, terrified they would be cut off if it was discovered that one of the kids had a paper route or some similar infraction.

For all the earlier talk of revolution, home relief under TERA was surprisingly similar to old-style public welfare, which is not to say that TERA organizers were insincere. Rather, the failure to match actions with words showed the stubbornness of old convictions. Home relief was founded on the premise that, if given the opportunity, even productive men and women would surrender to temptation and settle into a life on the dole.

Hopkins himself thought it would undermine the work ethic, convinced that "if a man keeps beating a path to the welfare office to get a grocery order he will gradually learn the way and it will be pretty hard to get him off that path."[18] Individuals were at risk, but if the will to work was compromised on a large enough scale, so was the future of the country. Such were the corrupting powers of charity! With so much at stake, TERA officials felt beholden to monitor their welfare clients, protecting both the American work ethic and the public treasury.

People receiving home relief, meanwhile, bristled at the supervision that reached into every room of the house but was most pronounced in the kitchen. TERA's decision to give help "in kind" was meant to diminish the appearance of a traditional money-based dole. However, it also helped control what TERA clients were eating. In some areas, including New York City, "pantry snoopers" accompanied women to the market to confirm that all parties (both shopper and shopkeeper) were complying with TERA's marketing guidelines. More prying took place in the kitchen itself, where investigators lifted pot covers and peered into iceboxes on the lookout for dietary violations.

As resentment smoldered, social workers began to question the wisdom of so much government meddling. A very public critique that ran in the *New York Times* sized up the dangers. "By our grocery-ticket dole," it began, "our bags of coal, our bundles of clothing, our rent vouchers, we have taken from people the right to manage their own lives."[19] The result of giving help "in kind" was more humiliation, people shamed into thinking they were incapable of doing the job on their own. Though no member of the family was completely safe from the long arms of TERA, supervision in all matters culinary was aimed directly at homemakers. Told what to cook, they were also told where to shop. With their food tickets good only at TERA-appointed stores, women were effectively barred from their corner grocers and sent on treks to unfamiliar merchants. Veteran homemakers, women who knew where the bargains were, not only resented the intrusion but were sure they could squeeze more out of their relief allowances by shopping at stores of their own choosing. By 1934, Hopkins, too, was having doubts about TERA's role as a dietary watchdog. Unsure of which was more damaging, "a lack of vitamins or complete surrender of choice," he abandoned the idea of grocery orders, replacing them with cash. If work was the best kind of help a person could receive, money was second, a lesson he carried to his next job as the director of federal relief under President Roosevelt.[20]

TWO YEARS INTO TERA, New Yorkers were still languishing on food allowances that were far short of adequate. One reason was the opposition put up by local welfare officials, the people in charge of putting those allowances into practice. Though created by the state, TERA was in fact a partnership between state and local governments, the first dependent on the second for cooperation. (Early on, Hopkins had chosen not to enforce TERA's welfare standards, adopting instead a policy of "education and persuasion.") The money to pay for TERA likewise came from both state and town treasuries, the price tag more or less split between them. Welfare officers in many of those towns proved unpersuadable. Comfortable with the old standards, officials with decades on the job felt that a four-dollar food allowance had always been good enough and saw no compelling reason to raise it. In rural districts, officers mistakenly assumed that farm families could provide their own eggs, chicken, fruit, and vegetables, and trimmed budgets based on food that did not exist. Others argued that local living standards had always been low, and that it was wrong for TERA clients to be dining on foods that the officers themselves could not afford. Then again, cooperation was not always a matter of choice. On the contrary, even with help from the state, adequate food relief was beyond the means of many communities, making compliance impossible. Powerless to do otherwise, officials who accepted the new standards were obliged to cut budgets already at minimum levels. Reports of slow starvation began filtering into TERA headquarters. "The amount allowed for food is inadequate for all families," one of them stated:

> *In addition to insufficient milk, there is no family which has had a sufficient amount of vegetables, either fresh or canned, including tomatoes, leafy or root vegetables.*
>
> *Vegetables which may be eaten raw were used only in a very few families and in small amounts.*
>
> *There are few families which have had a sufficient amount of potatoes.*
>
> *There is no family which has had a sufficient amount of fruit and few families have had any dried fruit.*
>
> *There is no family which has used a sufficient amount of dark cooked or breakfast cereals or dark bread . . .*
>
> *There is no family which has not used some eggs, but few families have had a sufficient number.*

Of the thirty families studied, the only foods eaten in relative abundance were macaroni and cooking oil.[21]

Exhilarated by the newness of what they were attempting, Hopkins and his top people shared an energizing esprit de corps. But novelty had drawbacks too. Having no precedents to lean on and no established relief standards to refer to, when TERA gave money for rent or to pay doctors' bills, it was forced to rely on educated guesswork. With so many people dependent on TERA, the vagueness about how much to give was a part of the job that rattled Hopkins. On one front, however, TERA could proceed with confidence. Food standards, unlike any other budget item, were *scientifically* determined, backed up by principles that never changed and that applied to everyone. However, not even science could account for all the variables that people introduced to the equation. Among them was the willingness of tens of thousands of women to follow the standards.

A home cook who had never heard of calories or vitamins, who was reluctant to take advice from strangers—and government strangers no less—required more than a pamphlet from the welfare office to accept the new food science. That it went against women's inclinations only added to their doubts. If the baby was crying for food, would a plate of cabbage stop her tears? In place of cabbage and carrots, women invested in pasta, rice, and bread, foods that satisfied an immediate need but left the children malnourished. To better educate those women and help close the nutrition deficit, home economists from around the state organized nutrition and cooking classes, staged cooking demonstrations, and went door-to-door as "visiting housekeepers" dispensing on-the-spot advice.

In collaboration with local welfare offices, home economists like Rose and Van Rensselaer worked as messengers, interpreting the government's advice and presenting it in practical terms women could appreciate. Where the TERA investigator was someone to be feared, visiting housekeepers were received as allies. Women once resistant to the gospel preached by home economists signed up for nutrition classes, anxious to know why their children were listless and pale. They attended lectures on wise food buying at the local church and formed neighborhood cooking classes. On leaving the welfare office, they picked up mimeographed recipes like the ones prepared by Cornell, read the department's nutrition bulletins, and sent in letters asking for information on topics ranging from the mechanics of digestion to methods of food preservation. This letter from a home-maker wondering about healthy ways to combine foods hints at the newly awakened desire for food knowledge:

*I am very interested in nutrition. I do not understand calories or vitamins, just what they are. I understand foods change when taken into the stomach but what I want to know is this: What foods go together . . . ? What is the difference in the stomach if coffee is mixed with milk before drinking or a cup of black coffee and a glass of milk taken separately. . . . I have seven children at home and I am continually studying what to feed [them] for [the] best results. . . . Milk I understand is the best food but does it not sometimes change to a harmful food with certain conditions of the stomach . . . ? There is so much I do not understand.*[22]

For home economists, an opportunity presented itself. Women who thought of their profession as a calling, who believed in the revolutionary possibilities of home economics but until now had reached only a modest audience, saw their stock rising. The public was ready to learn, and home economists would take full advantage of, a story that had already begun to play out on a national scale.

# Chapter 6

ERBERT HOOVER LIKED to say that the gourmets of the world should forget Paris and go to Iowa, advice that said more about his politics than his food preferences. As a grown man, Hoover looked back on his Iowa childhood as a kind of Eden on the prairie, unspoiled countryside populated by sturdy, Bible-reading men and women. Set loose to explore the natural world, ten-year-old "Bert" fished, hunted with a slingshot, and swam in a mud-bottomed pond, but like everyone else on the farm, he worked too. To Hoover's profound approval, self-sufficiency was the farmer's way of life. Whatever the family needed, it produced, each farm its own soap company, carpet factory, flour mill, and cannery. For Hoover, Iowa farmhouse cooking was a cuisine of self-reliance, the Sunday meals of ham and cornbread edible testimony to the values he saw as America's bedrock. The barrels and jars of winter provisions put up by farm women every fall were, in Hoover's own words, "social security itself."

The food that Hoover admired so much in theory was not necessarily the food he chose to eat. In his pre-presidential life as a mining executive, Hoover had crisscrossed the globe, making the rounds of Europe's top eating spots. By the time he returned to the United States, he had developed a worldly appreciation for Continental dining, which was also shared by his wife, Lou Henry Hoover. When Hoover was appointed secretary of commerce, the couple bought a mansion and immediately began throwing parties. Lou earned a reputation as a charming and generous hostess, while the Hoovers' cook, Mary Rattley, became famous among the political set for her oyster soufflés and fish with cucumber sauce.

As the country's most visible dinner hosts, President and Mrs. Hoover raised their hospitality standards to levels previously unknown in the White House. Within days of Hoover's taking office, Washington observers declared an end to "simple fare" at the presidential dinner table—Coolidge was known for his taste for plain food—and the start of a new, more elevated dining era. The change was regarded with some amount of uneasiness. As one White House watcher described it, "President Hoover is an eater. A large, discriminating eater. He might even be called, in the milder sense of the word, a gourmet."[1] Dishes with unpronounceable names that the couple had discovered on their travels were introduced to the White House menu, causing anxiety for a kitchen staff unfamiliar with foreign cooking. (If the cook was ever at a loss, the head housekeeper would consult with Mrs. Hoover, who provided the kitchen with detailed cooking instructions.) Ingredients used in the Hoover kitchen were often imported or out of season but were always the best available. Unsurprisingly, the Hoovers' entertaining costs far exceeded the White House budget. To cover the bill, the Hoovers took the unusual step of making up the difference from their own substantial bank account.

The style in which the Hoovers fed their guests confirmed the impression of opulence. A grand affair under any administration, a formal dinner during the Hoovers' tenure was occasion to unlock the White House treasure chest. The dining room was awash in gold. Running down the center of the table, a gilt-edged mirror purchased by President Monroe was flanked by gold-plated dishes, forks, knives, and spoons. The table was lit by many-branched golden candelabra and decorated with tall gold epergnes, ornate bowls filled with luscious fruit. At the inaugural dinner, even Mrs. Hoover was encased in gold, greeting dignitaries in a gleaming gold brocade gown.

At the head of the table, Hoover was like a nervous schoolboy at his own birthday party, the focus of attention but too overwhelmed to join in the festivities. Known as abnormally reserved, Hoover was a reluctant politician who hated the glad-handing and similar tasks required of his office. At the table, he was more comfortable as a listener than a talker, his reticence easily interpreted as aloofness. Of course, formality was expected at state dinners, but even when the Hoovers dined alone, their meals were taken in the state dining room, the president attired in a black dinner jacket. A row of butlers in tails and white ties stood at attention, all of them the same height—as Mrs. Hoover insisted—with the exception of the towering head butler, Alonzo Fields. Not even Fields, however, was permitted to speak to the president unless spoken to. When the tables were cleared, the men were under strict orders to prevent the silverware from clinking against the china. To people in the Hoovers' orbit, particularly those who worked in the White House, the rigid etiquette seemed to confirm the president's remoteness, which was ironic for a man known as "the great humanitarian." More forgiving observers, however, said that Hoover was just as compassionate as before, only now the real Herbert Hoover was hidden behind a front of "presidential dignity." As his term progressed and the economy continued to unravel, the first couple's lavish entertainments added to the perception that the president was out of touch with the travails of average Americans during a time of national crisis. He considered scaling back but, on reflection, decided against it. Casting himself in the role of unflinching leader, he resolved to carry on as part of his "business as usual" policy.

Attitude was key. In Hoover's analysis, the panic on Wall Street had prompted consumer hysteria that in turn had hurt

American manufacturers, causing further panic, and so on in a never-ending loop. As the head of state, Hoover felt it was his job to break the cycle of anxiety by projecting a confident demeanor. At the same time, Hoover was opposed to any program that could undermine what he saw as the core American values of individualism, self-help, and local voluntarism. On the grounds that greater government involvement would endanger the American spirit of charity—"something infinitely valuable" in Hoover's judgment—his main vehicle for helping the unemployed offered them nothing more concrete than government enthusiasm. Founded in October 1931, the President's Emergency Committee for Employment obeyed the central tenet that help for the unemployed was a local responsibility. As a result, PECE devoted itself to the coordination and mobilization of local relief efforts, its successes trumpeted by a vigorous public relations machine.

In his past life as a relief administrator, Hoover had never been afraid to jump on a train and travel to the heart of a crisis. True, the sight of human suffering had always rattled him, particularly the suffering of children, but at no time had that stopped him from getting close enough to any disaster to make a firsthand appraisal. During his presidency, however, Hoover steered clear of the breadlines and employment bureaus. He never toured Appalachia or Mississippi or interviewed one of the newly unemployed. Bizarrely, the investigative instincts that had served him so well as an administrator seemed to elude him as president. In place of making on-the-scene assessments, for information on the jobless he turned to PECE members, visiting businessmen, and allied politicians, almost all of them Republican. Based largely on their reporting, the president decided that Americans needed to step up their own attempts at charity, one neighbor helping the next. The government can't do all of it, he explained to reporters. And besides, he added, "Nobody is actually starving."[2] A claim often repeated by Hoover and his supporters, "No one has starved" became the fallback response to all those "purveyors of gloom" hawking their grim statistics and dire predictions. Proof that a government dole still was unnecessary, it also justified Hoover's refusal to grant federal relief.

Nevertheless, Hoover's optimism was belied by reports that began to appear in newspapers across the country. In Toledo, Ohio, a young mother walked into a diner, holding her two-year-old son:

> *"Just some milk and cereal for the baby," she told the waiter with the greasy apron. "That will be a dime won't it? I'm not hungry." After the child had eaten, she picked the last dime from her shabby purse, walked out into the wintry night and collapsed.[3]*

The woman survived, but others, it appeared, were too far gone. In Hartford, a thirty-seven-year-old "work dodger" was discovered unconscious. The man was promptly taken to a hospital, where doctors tried to revive him, but "his resistance was too greatly undermined by lack of nourishment."[4] In New Orleans, a seventy-six-year-old man collapsed in a soup kitchen. His last words were "I never asked anyone for help." His death certificate read "heart attack," but welfare workers said he died of starvation.

Faced with growing evidence of a health crisis across the United States, Hoover asked the surgeon general to prepare a report comparing sickness and mortality in the first five months of both 1928 and 1931. The president could not have hoped for better news. According to the country's chief doctor, the economic crisis seemed to have had no adverse effects on America's health. Both tuberculosis deaths and infant mortality had actually dropped, and influenza rates were unusually low.[5] The report gave Hoover permission to follow his conscience. That October, in place of a federal relief program, Hoover founded the President's Organization on Unemployment Relief, a committee of businessmen led by Walter Gifford, president of AT&T, which was assigned to raise money for local charities. Using every form of media at its disposal, POUR began a massive fund-raising campaign. Through advertisements in newspapers and magazines, on radio and city billboards, POUR appealed to the public's sense of civic responsibility with slogans like "I Will Share" and "Of Course We Can Do It." The American public, however, was unswayed. A man who liked to keep his fingertips on the numbers, Hoover could see that the drives were earning diminishing returns. Conservative allies nevertheless assured him that funds were sufficient to help the unemployed through the winter. Hoover listened to his advisers and, ignoring the numbers, stayed on course with his no-relief policy into the election year of 1932.

Early that year, the starvation question seemed to receive a definitive answer. Its source was the chief statistician of the Metropolitan Life Insurance Company. In January, after tabulating the company's mortality records, Dr. Louis Dublin discovered that the nation was in excellent health. In spite of the Depression, the basic needs of policyholders for food, clothing, and shelter had been well met.[6] What's more, the weight-loss program imposed by the Depression may have been exactly what the country needed. "As a people," Dublin explained,

> *we are given normally to overfeeding, and this has led to much trouble, as every physician knows. I would not be surprised if, under the present conditions of enforced moderation, many have enjoyed better health than ever before.[7]*

With regard to starvation, the doctor was unambiguous. Dublin had found "no evidence at all that anybody in these United States is starving," news that should hearten worried Americans.[8]

Dublin's "no starvation" announcement appeared in an article he had written for the social work magazine *Better Times*. Where the man on the street may have taken the doctor at his word, the welfare professionals who were the publication's main readers had seen enough of the Depression to question the accuracy of his assertion. Aware of the controversy, the editors of *Better Times* offered its readers this challenge: "Is Dr. Dublin right? Is there no evidence of starvation? BETTER TIMES invites those who have the evidence to cite it." The answer came in an article published that April. According to hospital records, in 1931, ninety-five people in New York City had been diagnosed with starvation and, of those, twenty had died from lack of food. And this was aside from the more widespread problem of malnutrition, the slow physical decline brought on by insufficient food that so often ended in premature death.[9]

Articles like this one helped inform a debate then taking place in Washington. Despite Hoover's no-relief policy, congressional Democrats and progressive Republicans, convinced of the need for federal relief, introduced bills in both the House and Senate to give as much as $250 million to help the unemployed. Hearings for the bills included testimony from a long line of social workers, labor leaders, unemployed miners, and so on, all bearing witness to the dire conditions in Philadelphia, Detroit, Chicago, Appalachia, and Mississippi cotton country. In case anyone believed these were merely localized conditions, the socialist journalist Oscar Ameringer recounted his recent experiences on a cross-country journey:

> *In the State of Washington I was told that the forest fires raging in that region all summer and fall were caused by unemployed timber workers and bankrupt farmers in an endeavor to earn a few honest dollars as fire fighters. The last thing I saw on the night I left Seattle was numbers of women searching for scraps of food in the refuse piles of the principal market of that city. A number of Montana citizens told me of thousands of bushels of wheat left in the fields uncut on account of its low price*

*that hardly paid for harvesting. In Oregon I saw thousands of bushels of apples rotting in the orchards. Only absolutely flawless apples were still salable, at from 40 to 50 cents a box containing 200 apples. At the same time, there are millions of children who, on account of their parents, will not eat one apple this winter. . . . I talked to one man in a restaurant in Chicago. He told me of his experience in raising sheep. He said that he had killed 3,000 sheep this fall and thrown them down the canyon, because it had cost $1.10 to ship a sheep, and then he would get less than a dollar for it. He said he could not afford to feed the sheep, and he would not let them starve, so he just cut their throats and threw them down the canyon. The roads of the West and Southwest teem with hungry hitchhikers. The camp fires of the homeless are seen along every railroad track. I saw men, women, and children walking over the hard roads. Most of them were tenant farmers who had lost their all in the late slump in wheat and cotton. Between Clarksville and Russellville, Ark., I picked up a family. The woman was hugging a dead chicken under a ragged coat. When I asked her where she had procured the fowl, first she told me she had found it dead in the road, and then added in grim humor, "They promised me a chicken in the pot, and now I got mine."*[10]

Despite accounts like Ameringer's, when relief measures came to a vote, they were blocked by a coalition of conservative Democrats and Republicans.

By early spring of 1932, however, doubts were beginning to creep into the minds of Hoover's political backers. Facing intense pressure, the president decided that relief for the unemployed had become unavoidable, though he needed to find some method of giving it that preserved his conservative principles. Above all, the federal government could give no support in the form of money. Hoover and his allies found the perfect alternative in the Federal

Farm Board. Founded by Hoover in 1929 to support agricultural prices, the board had purchased millions of bushels of wheat in a failing effort to help wheat farmers. Now the slowly moldering grain was being stored in silos across the Midwest. In a plan devised by the Red Cross and wheat state politicians, the board donated the grain to the Red Cross, which then shipped it to mills across the Great Plains. The resulting white flour was packed into twenty-four-pound sacks with the following inscription:

*BLEACHED*
*24 lbs.*
*MILLED FROM*
*GOVERNMENT OWNED WHEAT*
*By Authority of*
*Act of Congress*
*FLOUR*
*DISTRIBUTED BY*
*THE AMERICAN RED CROSS*
*NOT TO BE SOLD*[11]

Beginning in March 1932, local government and private charity agencies across the country were encouraged to apply for shipments of Red Cross flour. Aid workers in Los Angeles estimated that they would need twenty-five railroad cars of flour per month to feed the city's hungry. After the first six carloads arrived in early April, the flour was off-loaded by a team of unemployed workers and distributed to local welfare agencies, the Salvation Army, and the YWCA. A portion was taken by the city's parent-teacher association to be used in its free lunch program. To make the most of government flour, many schools changed their menu plans, using less store-bought bread and replacing it with meat pies and hot biscuits.[12]

The Red Cross expected that families given government flour would use it to make bread. They were surprised to discover that large numbers of American homemakers had forgotten how to bake. To help fill the knowledge gap, the Red Cross distributed pamphlets with simple recipes for baking-powder biscuits, kneaded biscuits, muffins, gingerbread, oatmeal, and drop cookies. Some communities opened their own bakeries, where they trained unemployed workers in bread-baking skills. Down South, however, flour distribution led to familiar claims of discrimination, as whites received flour with no questions asked, but blacks were required to work on road repair projects before they were considered worthy. The Red Cross chose not to investigate. Still, by July 1932, it had distributed more than thirty million bushels of wheat to millions of unemployed Americans in more than 75 percent of the country's counties. Hoover and the Red Cross touted the success of the program, but as observers pointed out, those impressive numbers were actually an illustration of the breadth and depth of the economic crisis.[13]

———————

THE RELIEF DEBATES in Washington were driven by concern for the unemployed. Behind that concern, however, lurked fear of what the growing numbers of jobless and hungry Americans might do if the situation continued. How long would they tolerate empty stomachs before they were driven to act? In the hills of Kentucky, coal miners told reporters they would steal before hearing their children cry for bread. After a riot over relief in Chicago, a pastor explained, "I can't tell a hungry man to be patient." In a coal district of Oklahoma, three hundred gaunt miners and their families marched into the town of Henryetta. After a brief prayer, they stormed local grocery stores, demanding food; the merchants meekly acquiesced. In Washington, testifying before yet another committee, Edward McGrady of the American Federation of Labor told senators that if nothing was done and starvation continued "the doors of revolution are going to be thrown wide open." In

fact, in a number of industrial cities Communists had already provoked uprisings, when all the protesters really wanted was bread.[14]

Actually, as McGrady and the senators well knew, Communists were behind some of the largest protest movements in cities from Boston to Los Angeles. In Moscow, Soviet leaders had
read the onset of the Great Depression as a sign that the world-
wide capitalist system had entered its final collapse. Determined
to push it over the edge, in early 1931 they instructed the Communist Party of the USA to organize a series of urban hunger
marches. Led by the Unemployed Councils, a group organized
by the CPUSA to guide the "struggles" of unemployed workers,
the marchers listened to Communist orators and carried banners
decorated with slogans like "Don't Starve, Fight!" The marches
generally culminated at city hall, where demonstrators demanded
to meet with the mayor. When a cordon of police denied them
entry, protests often turned bloody, with officers wading into the
crowd with nightsticks while protesters answered with fists and
bricks. Afterward, both sides could claim success: the police jailed
a good number of violent "Reds," while the Communists earned
front-page stories. The success of these local demonstrations led to
the organization of the National Hunger March at the end of 1931,
when delegations from around the country converged on Washington. Despite predictions of widespread violence, the march
ended quietly, as Washington's police chief, Pelham Glassford,
negotiated the marchers' peaceful entry into the capital and allowed them to present their petitions to Congress.

Three months later in Detroit, one of the country's most eco-
nomically troubled cities, another hunger march ended in tragedy.
Following a sharp drop in auto sales, Henry Ford had fired thousands of his Detroit-area workers. At the same time, he refused to
donate to any of the local relief organizations that were helping
feed and house his ex-employees. To protest, and to try to squeeze
some money out of Henry Ford, the Unemployed Councils

organized a hunger march on March 7, 1932 (the same day that Hoover signed the wheat distribution bill), from Detroit to Ford's River Rouge plant in nearby Dearborn. At the Dearborn city line, the marchers, a mix of laid-off Ford workers and young Communists, were met by hundreds of Dearborn policemen and Ford security guards, all of them armed. When the marchers refused an order to stop, a shot was fired from the Dearborn side, the start of a running battle in which four protesters were killed and fifty more were injured. (The injured were later manacled to their hospital beds and placed under arrest.) While Ford blamed the violence on the City of Detroit for allowing the march to take place, local newspapers accused the Dearborn police of using their guns on unarmed citizens. In Washington, it was possible to excuse the violence because it involved Communists, enemies worthy of the most extreme response. However, President Hoover and the Republicans would soon find themselves facing the challenge of a far larger march right in their own backyard.

IN 1930, A man named Walter Waters lost his job as assistant superintendent of a cannery near Portland, Oregon. A veteran of the Great War, Walters had returned eleven years earlier from Europe to be greeted by parades and homecoming banquets. After his discharge from service, however, he found work elusive, bouncing from job to low-paying job in his native Idaho. Fed up, one day he hitchhiked to Washington State, got a job as a harvest hand, and started a new life. He soon married and moved to Portland, where the couple had two children. He found a job in the cannery and slowly worked his way up to better-paying positions. When he lost his job, the family turned to its savings and Walker hit the streets, looking for work. When the money ran out, the family's personal belongings one by one found their way to the pawnshop, until they had nothing left but a few clothes.

The family survived thanks to the patience of their landlord, a veteran himself, the charity of neighbors, and food relief from the city.

As he traveled around Portland, Waters ran into many men in the same position. Years later, when he wrote his autobiography, he recorded his impression of those fellow job-hunters: "men in threadbare clothing pacing the sidewalk in soleless shoes, on their faces the same look, part of hope, part of bewilderment, as they searched for a chance to earn a few dollars at honest work."[15] Many of them were down-on-their-luck veterans like himself: "They had fought, so they had been told a few years before, 'to save the nation'; they had fought, it now seemed, only in order to have a place in which to starve."[16] As they waited in employment offices, in relief lines, and along the city's Skid Row, their conversations often turned to the question of the "bonus" for World War I veterans. In 1924, Congress had voted (over Coolidge's veto) for the World War Adjusted Compensation Act, which was meant to make up the difference between a soldier's pay during wartime and what he would have made in civilian life. The maximum a veteran could hope to receive was $625. The catch, however, was that this bonus was not scheduled to be paid until 1945. For men hunkered down in the trenches of the Great Depression, that seemed a long time to wait; $600 could make a huge difference to the life of a hungry and jobless veteran. Some Democratic politicians agreed.

Since 1929, Congressman Wright Patman of Texas had campaigned for a bill to amend the Compensation Act to pay out the bonuses immediately. By early 1932, it looked like the bill might finally come up for a vote, against the strenuous opposition of the president, almost all Republicans, and even many Democrats (including Governor Roosevelt). Portland's veterans' association asked all its members to sign petitions and write to politicians to help secure the vote. Walter Waters was a little more canny about the ways of Washington: "Our only hope was in following the successful tactics of Big Business; when its representatives wanted something from Congress, they went to it personally and said so."[17] He stood up in veterans' meetings and suggested that Portland veterans send a delegation to Washington to directly lobby senators and congressmen. Initially, the men were unconvinced and trusted their government to do the right thing. But in Washington, politicians from both parties saw the bonus bill as a license to print money without the backing of gold or bond issues. On May 6, 1932, the House Ways and Means Committee voted to permanently shelve the bonus bill. Four days later, Portland's veterans agreed to send a delegation of 250 men under strict military discipline to the nation's capital. That same day, they headed down to the rail yards to embark on their journey across the United States.

As with all armies, the first and ongoing challenge of the "Bonus Army" was to secure provisions. The men arrived at the yards with no food and only a few dollars between them, hoping to catch a freight train heading east. While most of the troop slept in empty freight cars for the night, Waters and some of his comrades went scavenging and found a few greasy spoons that were still open. The owners were sympathetic to their cause and willing to donate coffee and bread. By jumping freights, cadging rides on trucks, and foraging for food, the men gradually made their way across the country, taking ten days to reach St. Louis. When they entered a new town, the marchers often staged impromptu parades, passing the hat to onlookers to raise money for the next leg of their journey. In East St. Louis, Illinois, however, they hit a roadblock at the Baltimore and Ohio freight yards. Railway officials refused to let the men board empty eastbound freight cars. In response, the Oregon veterans blocked the tracks, bringing one of the nation's most important freight lines to a standstill. The police were the first on the scene, followed by reporters; when the governor called in six companies of the Illinois National Guard, the Bonus Marchers became national news. Finally, the local sheriff rounded up a fleet of trucks to ship the men east. Let them be another sheriff's problem, not his. Meanwhile, in Texas, Florida, Maine, Michigan, California, and dozens of other states, thousands of veterans suffering through hard times had read about the Oregon marchers, and they, too, hit the road for the nation's capital. By May 29, when Walter Waters and his men finally made it to Washington, more contingents were on their way, some as large as 1,500 men, with a few wives and children in tow as well.

Washington's police chief, Pelham Glassford, had done his best to keep the protesters from entering the city, but now that they were there he felt he had no choice but to help them find food and a place to stay. Most were sent to camp at the far side of the Anacostia River, with a view of the Capitol building just over the trees. The site was little more than a tidal flat that turned to mud when it rained and stank from the sewage in the river. Others found makeshift lodgings in buildings slated for demolition nearer the Capitol. As one reporter described them, the men were visibly at the end of their ropes, "close enough to starvation to know what it means for themselves and their families."[18]

The veterans' camp became something of a local spectacle. Many of the Washingtonians who came to view it were sympathetic to the veterans' cause. Among them was the wealthy socialite Evalyn Walsh McLean, owner of the Hope Diamond and estranged wife of the owner of the *Washington Post*. Late one night, Mrs. McLean found Glassford, and the pair drove to a nearby Childs restaurant. Mrs. McLean bought a thousand sandwiches and a thousand packs of cigarettes, while Glassford paid out of his own pocket for a thousand cups of coffee, all of which became breakfast for the Bonus marchers. Glassford also rounded up donations of four 150-pound turtles to make into turtle stew and 1,500 pounds of pork from the Dixie Barbecue Company. He called up the local National Guard barracks and found a half

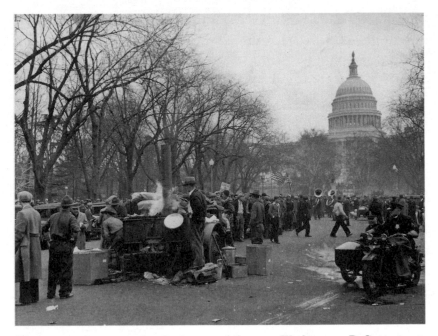

*Hunger marchers preparing food on a mobile stove, Washington, D.C.* (Authors'
collection)

dozen U.S. Army rolling kitchens that the veterans could use to
cook their meals. Meanwhile, the marchers began to construct a
makeshift, "rag-and-tin-can city" on the Anacostia Flats, scavenging lumber, furniture, old cars, and anything else that could
be used as shelter.

During the first weeks of the Bonus Army's encampment, Chief
Glassford tried to find some organization that would help feed the
veterans, but the city government and various veterans' groups refused. He went to the Red Cross, but it agreed to donate only a
small amount of flour and no milk for the camp's children. Glassford had better luck with local sports fans, who organized a professional boxing match that raised $2,700 to buy supplies. Finally,
however, he had to give primary responsibility for feeding the men,
now numbering roughly twenty thousand, to Walter Waters and
the other Bonus Army leaders. The feeding system they organized

was along the lines of the U.S. Army's Quartermaster Corps. The men were fed twice a day, early in the morning and again around 4 or 5 p.m. For Waters, finding supplies was a constant challenge:

> *We managed during the entire time to furnish bread and cof-*
> *fee as a minimum and never once failed. The rest of the menu*
> *varied from turtle soup to boiled grits. Only by the narrowest*
> *margin on one or two days in July was sufficient food secured*
> *to prevent a foodless day. Never was there food in plenty. "This*
> *camp oughta be called 'No Seconds,'" was a remark that sums*
> *up the entire food situation. One day there would have been no*
> *"firsts" if a manufacturer in New York had not supplied fifteen*
> *hundred pounds of meat that was sent down by airplane.*[19]

Instead of army mess kits, for plates the veterans used old newspapers. On good days, the main dish was "slumgullion," a term originally coined during the California gold rush days to describe the watery mixture of mud and gravel left over from the mining process. During the war, it became slang for army beef stew. Serving one hundred soldiers, the army recipe called for twenty-five pounds of beef and twenty pounds of potatoes, both cubed and then stewed with four pounds of onions, the broth thickened with a pound of flour. The men were unanimous in praising it as better than anything they had received in the breadline, sopping it up with bread from Ottenberg's, a local Jewish bakery.

During the first weeks of their Washington stay, the majority of veterans spent their days in camp, playing cards, singing army songs, and composing ditties:

> *Mellon pulled the whistle,*
> *Hoover rang the bell,*
> *Wall Street gave the signal*
> *And the country went to Hell!*[20]

While the men bided their time, their leaders pressed the case for early payment of the bonus with senators, congressmen, the vice president, and any other politician who would listen, and many did. One who did not was Hoover. Determined that no ragtag group of protesters, even those who had served their country, would disrupt the dignity of his office, the president refused to engage with them. Moreover, he was increasingly convinced that the Bonus Army was actually a Communist-instigated movement. (There were certainly Communists among the veterans, but they were a minority and were kept isolated by Bonus Army leaders.) In any case, Hoover had a campaign to run and was either busy preparing for the Republican convention or, on weekends, resting in his camp in the Virginia mountains.

In the absence of clear leadership from the White House, the situation outside its gates deteriorated as the summer progressed. The food supply for the Bonus Army was running low, and children living in the camps showed signs of malnutrition. After Congress adjourned in mid-July, the army turned its attentions on the president, who steadfastly refused a meeting. After weeks of noisy pickets and a few attempts by veterans to sneak into the White House, Hoover and the city commissioners decided that they had had enough of the Bonus Marchers. On July 21, Waters was told that they must leave the downtown buildings where some had camped, return the army's rolling kitchens, and be out of Anacostia Flats by August 4. The veterans wanted to stay put—they had nowhere else to go—and planned to find a permanent encampment on private land. Meanwhile, the U.S. Army's chief of staff, General Douglas MacArthur, was convinced that the protesters were insurgents bent on revolution and had begun to quietly move tanks and other weapons into the city. Waters thought he could get an extension, but on July 28 his men received word that they must immediately evacuate downtown buildings. As the police watched, the men filed out peacefully, until a sudden scuffle broke out. A policeman panicked and shot two veterans, killing one and mortally wounding the other.

On word of the shootings, Hoover decided that Glassford had lost control of the situation and ordered the U.S. Army to clear the veterans from downtown Washington. General MacArthur leaped at the invitation. Under his command, two hundred saber-wielding cavalrymen, five tanks, and trucks of infantrymen with bayonets rolled down Pennsylvania Avenue as crowds gathered to watch. When soldiers reached the camp, they were met by rocks, and hurled teargas bombs in return. As clouds of teargas engulfed the spectators, soldiers chased the veterans from the row of abandoned buildings that had been their temporary home. The men fled toward Anacostia, followed by U.S. Army troops. At this point, General MacArthur unilaterally decided that his job was to expel the Bonus Army from Washington. When the soldiers paused at the Anacostia Bridge, a messenger caught up to MacArthur with word from the president: the soldiers must not evict the veterans (now numbering seven thousand men, women, and children) from Anacostia. Shortly after the messenger left, the general ordered his men to storm the camp. Under the glare of spotlights, soldiers marched across the bridge and into the jumble of improvised shelters, tossing more teargas bombs and setting shacks ablaze. Veterans and their families grabbed their belongings and ran. Anacostia was soon in flames, the vast orange glow visible from the White House.

IN THE AFTERMATH of the July 28 rout from Washington, editorial pages around the country showed their support for Hoover's handling of the Bonus Army, blaming the violence on the Communists, the (Democratic) politicians who lured the veterans to Washington with false hopes, and the veterans themselves. Back in New York, however, Governor Roosevelt saw the burning of

Anacostia as an instance of political suicide. Sitting up in his bed on the following morning, the *New York Times* open in front of him, Roosevelt told an aide there was no need to drag Anacostia into the campaign. The reporters had done it for them. "Why didn't Hoover offer the men coffee and sandwiches instead of turning . . . Doug MacArthur loose?"[21] As Americans read the newspaper articles and watched newsreel footage of the U.S. Army bearing down on poor and defenseless veterans, public sentiment began to peel away from the president. His treatment of the Bonus Army became a symbol of everything that was wrong with the country, a sentiment encapsulated in the E. Y. "Yip" Harburg song "Brother, Can You Spare a Dime?":

> *They used to tell me I was building a dream*
> *And so I followed the mob.*
> *When there was earth to plow or guns to bear,*
> *I was always there, right on the job.*
>
> *They used to tell me I was building a dream*
> *With peace and glory ahead—*
> *Why should I be standing in line,*
> *Just waiting for bread?*
>
> *Once I built a railroad, I made it run,*
> *Made it race against time.*
> *Once I built a railroad, now it's done—*
> *Brother, can you spare a dime?*[22]

By the time the Bonus Army left Washington, the presidential campaign of 1932 had slightly more than three months left. Fixated on the principle that each man is his brother's keeper, Hoover was unwavering on the subject of relief. In a major speech, he promised that "no man, woman or child shall go hungry or unsheltered through the coming winter," insisting that local charities could manage the job.

Roosevelt's 1932 platform was not all that different. Like the president, he would work for balanced budgets and was against the veterans' bonus. On the subject of federal relief, however, the two men diverged. Back in April, Roosevelt had given his famous "Forgotten Man" speech, accusing the current administration of worrying too much about propping up the banks, railroads, and corporations at the top of the economic pyramid while ignoring the people below. Roosevelt's critics, often rightly, accused the governor of speaking in "glittering generalities." A week before the election, however, he gave a speech that clearly expressed his vision of the federal government's role in relief:

> *This nation . . . owes a positive duty that no one shall be permitted to starve. This means that while the immediate responsibility for relief rests with local, public and private charity, in so far as these are inadequate the states must carry the burden, and whenever states are unable adequately to do so the Federal government owes the positive duty of stepping into the breach.*[23]

The aura of presidential dignity that Hoover had worked so hard to cultivate now eluded him. On the campaign trail he looked drawn, tired, and bereft of ideas, while Roosevelt exuded optimism. When the American people went to the polls on November 8, 1932, they overwhelmingly voted for Franklin Delano Roosevelt as their next president.

# Chapter 7

———•◦•———

LOUISE ARMSTRONG, A Chicago social worker, and her husband, Harry, a commercial artist, were unemployed and nearly broke. One by one, the city's banks were failing, and they were afraid theirs would be next. As an insurance policy, they kept a short stack of traveler's checks locked away in a safe deposit box. In the spring of 1932, with no prospects for future work in sight, they cashed them in and left Chicago, joining a larger exodus. During the 1930s, decades of "city drift" finally reversed itself as urban America looked to the countryside for salvation. With factories closing, young workers who had escaped the family farm during the boom years returned to the countryside and the old patterns of subsistence agriculture. Rather than join the breadline, unemployed executives gave up their city addresses and decamped with their families to weekend homes to wait out the crisis. The Armstrongs' rural retreat was a summer home in the town of Manistee, Michigan, on the eastern shore of Lake Michigan. That March they took a ferry across the lake, reopened their house, and lugged their old flivver out of the barn. They could live for cheap in Manistee, supplementing their larder with food from their garden and small orchard.

More than a hundred miles from Grand Rapids, the nearest real city, Manistee had little in common with the rural idyll depicted by the Michigan writer Della Lutes. Summers were short, while winters were long and bitterly cold. Near the lake, the soil was too sandy for large-scale farming. Farther inland, the terrain was marshy and rocky, unsuited to most crops, with the exception of cherries and apples. For a good thirty years the region's main "crop" had been timber. In the late nineteenth century, lumberjacks had swarmed Manistee's white pine and hardwood forests, sawing down trees that had been standing for more than four hundred years. The logs were hauled to local mills by horse and wagon, the lumber shipped to Chicago and other burgeoning cities. Manistee glittered with lumber wealth, the foundation of a local economy that also supported sawmills, shipping concerns, and, for nighttime entertainment, saloons. Manistee was known as a wide-open town, a lucrative stopover for glassware salesmen because lumbermen, when properly drunk, liked to smash their drinking vessels. Celebrations of a more subdued nature took place on the hill that overlooked town. Here, in mansions built on lumber fortunes, Manistee's leading citizens hired orchestras from Detroit and Chicago to play at their soirees. In 1900, the city population peaked at eighteen thousand, but the timber industry was already in decline. With the forest reduced to stumps (Armstrong thought the stumps looked like tombstones), the lumbermen began to move farther north and west. In 1920, a fire burned down the last of the big sawmills, spurring the exodus of hundreds of families and bringing the lumber era to a close. Manistee sputtered along, thanks mainly to the discovery of large, subterranean salt deposits. The Board of Commerce waged a campaign to attract new industries, but Manistee was too remote and transportation too expensive to make them profitable. Before the decade was over, the population had dropped to a little more than eight thousand, and any industries that remained were cutting jobs. By the time of the crash, Manistee had already been in decline for thirty years.

The Depression hit different parts of Manistee in different ways. In town, laid-off workers imagined what they would do if the situation got any worse. If it got bad enough, they would go down Main Street, smashing windows and grabbing what they needed if that would keep their wives and children from starving. In homes up on the hill, staunch Republicans thought prosperity was, indeed, "just around the corner." Only dimly aware of the desperate stories coming out of Chicago and Detroit, in 1932 they were shocked when one of Manistee's two banks failed overnight. Many lost their life's savings. For the first time in memory, they turned down the heat in their drafty mansions to cut back on expenses. With no money to pay college tuition, their children dropped out and moved home. Young people who expected to work in the family business were thrown into limbo waiting to see if jobs would return. Those with marriage plans put them on hold.

When conditions finally began to change, it was not in the way they expected. Much to their surprise, in November 1932, Franklin Delano Roosevelt carried not only the state but their own county in the presidential elections. The following March, with every radio in town tuned to his inauguration, Roosevelt promised "direct, vigorous, action" to bring back the economy and unify the nation's relief efforts. By the next afternoon, he had already begun to make good on his pledge to the American people, starting with a bank holiday to restore confidence in the nation's financial system. But amid the swirl of political activity that made up the first hundred days of the new administration, it took several months to open the taps for federal relief. In April, Harry Hopkins presented Roosevelt with a plan for federal relief that drew on his experience directing the Temporary Emergency Relief Administration back in New York. Like TERA, this program would also be temporary, lasting only until they could set up a works program. In the meantime, the federal government, in a historic first, would spend billions of dollars on direct relief for the American people. Roosevelt gave the plan his blessing, and in early May Congress passed the act that created the Federal Emergency Relief Administration. Roosevelt immediately appointed Harry Hopkins as director. The day after FERA opened its doors, Hopkins authorized the first federal grants to seven hard-hit states, including Michigan, but significant strings were attached. To receive federal money, state and local governments were required to contribute as well, and to set up their own network of relief offices. To ensure compliance, every relief organization would be regularly investigated and audited, down to the amount of money given for food in a town like Manistee, Michigan.

In late September 1933, Louise Armstrong received a visit from the son of Manistee's new Democratic congressman asking if what he had heard was true. Did she have a college degree and had she once been employed as a social worker in Chicago? The answer was yes on both counts, making Armstrong the only person with professional social work experience in the county. That was enough to qualify her for the job of running Manistee's new Emergency Relief Office.

During a decade of summer visits, Louise Armstrong's interactions with native Manisteeans had been mainly confined to tradesmen in town. As the new emergency relief director, she encountered hundreds of residents from every nook and cranny of the county. Those encounters became the raw material for Armstrong's *We Too Are the People,* her account of three years in the relief business. One of the job's surprises was the questions it elicited from friends and acquaintances who had managed to stay off relief rolls. As Armstrong discovered, these people had no clue about how relief worked and whom, exactly, it benefited. Part character study, part sociological report, and part administrative history, *We Too Are the People* illuminated the unique subculture that grew up around the relief office. The book's title was Armstrong's reminder that "relief cases" were full-blown individuals with families and personal histories just like everyone else. At the same time, part of her job as a social worker was sorting her clients according to type. It was standard professional practice for a 1930s social worker to classify people as either "high" or "low" types, a supposedly clinical designation based on their position in the social order. So, according to Armstrong, the businessmen who lived on the hill were made of high-grade material. Ethnically they were either "Americans" (descendants of French and English settlers) or Scandinavians. A lower grade of townspeople, mostly Poles, lived near the mills along the riverfront. Out in the countryside, American, Scandinavian, and German farmers—high grade—tended orchards full of sour cherry and apple trees. A community of Finns near the town of Keleva specialized in growing cucumbers, the harvest sent to nearby pickling factories. They were high grade too. At the north end of the county, families whom Armstrong describes as "hillbillies of the north"—very low grade—lived in shacks and farmhouses abandoned by their previous tenants. Native American Ottawa lived along the banks of the Manistee River and could be either high or low types, "just like any other people."[1]

———

MANISTEE'S CULINARY CULTURE reflected both the county's geography and its ethnic complexity. Fish was a mainstay of the local diet, primarily Lake Michigan whitefish and trout, bass, and perch from the region's many lakes and streams. Fish was cooked simply: boiled in salt water, fried, or made into a fish chowder, to which cooks added a selection of root vegetables such as potatoes, turnips, parsnips, and carrots. In winter, men cut holes into the ice and fished with spears and homemade lures filled with lead, which they dangled in the frigid water. They went after suckers, trout, and northern pike, a bony fish that was cut into steaks, dredged in flour, and fried. Suckers, like catfish, were bottom feeders. Women soaked them in brine until the bones had softened, at which point the entire fish, bones and all, was ground into a pungent paste used as a sandwich spread. Despite the availability of fresh fish, canned salmon was used liberally, the main ingredient in croquettes, casseroles, and the ever-popular salmon loaf made with bread crumbs, eggs, milk, and onion. Like most of rural Michigan, Manistee abounded in game, including deer, woodchuck, and beaver. Venison steaks fried with onions and eaten with homemade bread were considered gourmet fare. Squirrel was simmered until tender, the cooking liquid used to make gravy. A Manistee community cookbook from the 1930s includes a rabbit recipe in which the butchered animal is rolled in flour, covered with cream, dotted with butter, and baked.

The apple and cherry orchards in and around Manistee made the region ideal for raising honeybees. Many farmers kept their own bees, which they used for pollination, but bees could also be rented. Transported to the orchard in frames, they were released to do their work, returning to the hive when done. Honey, a by-product of all that pollinating, was often used along with sugar in cakes, cookies, and preserves. The following recipe is from the *Manistee County Pomona Grange Cook Book,* published in 1938:

CHOCOLATE CAKE

½ cup butter
¾ cup cocoa
½ cup hot water
1 cup sugar
3 teaspoons baking powder

1 cup honey

4 eggs

1 cup milk

2½ cups cake flour

Cream butter, sugar, honey and cocoa and add the hot water, beat well, then add well beaten eggs, flour, baking powder and milk. Bake in a moderate oven (350) for 40 to 50 minutes.[2]

———

Manistee was meat loaf country. Recipes for beef, pork, ham, liver, veal, and chicken meat loaf show up frequently in community cookbooks from Manistee and the surrounding counties. A close relative, pressed meat, was made from beef or chicken that had been boiled until falling off the bone, chopped fine, packed into a tin loaf pan, and weighted until it was dense enough to slice. Casseroles made from corn, noodles, beans, and potatoes made frequent appearances. A dish called "Spanish rice" (many dishes were identified as Spanish simply because they contained tomatoes) was a popular casserole made with fried ham, bacon, or salt pork, chopped onion, tomato, diced bell pepper, and boiled rice, all combined and baked or warmed on the stove top. Spanish rice was popular enough in Manistee to be a featured dish at "community meals" held by the local grange. Tart, spicy, and sweet, homemade pickles and relishes added an acidic spark to meals based around protein and starch.

Community cookbooks show the influence of German, Scandinavian, and Polish cooking on the local cuisine. German "coffee breads," herring salad, and liver sausage are a few of the German recipes in the *Manistee County Pomona Grange Cook Book*. Layered, custard-filled Swedish torte also makes an appearance. Women of Scandinavian descent shared their recipes for northern European rye breads made with buttermilk and caraway. Polish women contributed recipes for yeast-risen butter cookies called kolaczki.

⸺ ·•· ⸺

AS THE COUNTY'S new relief administrator, Louise Armstrong was handed FERA's rules and regulations, a large pile of forms, and money to hire caseworkers and rent a downtown office. By mid-October, less than three weeks after she was hired, Manistee's new Emergency Relief Office was up and running. Armstrong's immediate task was to get food as quickly as possible into the hands of the unemployed. The old and disabled, former charges of the county poor commission, made up her first day's applicants. Following their initial interview, like all other prospective clients they received a home visit from the FERA investigator to collect the facts and figures needed to determine the amount of relief dollars to be given. Investigators recorded the number and ages of family members and all household expenses, but they also asked if there was a mortgage on the house, if the family had a bank account, if money was owed to the grocer.

To help states determine the family's food needs, FERA distributed copies of Hazel Stiebeling's *Food Budgets for Nutrition and Production Programs,* a guide written for relief administrators that was based on *Diets at Four Levels of Nutrient Content and Cost.* On the assumption that relief would be temporary, the guide came with instructions to follow the least generous "Restricted Diet," intended only for emergencies. To help state relief workers make the necessary computations, *Food Budgets* was illustrated with detailed nutritional tables. The recommendations displayed in those tables, however, were provisional suggestions based on science that was still quickly evolving. The process of implementing them, moreover, introduced a host of variables into the dietary arithmetic. In Michigan alone, the money given to a family of five ranged from $1.80 to $5.00 a week, resulting in a culinary patchwork that

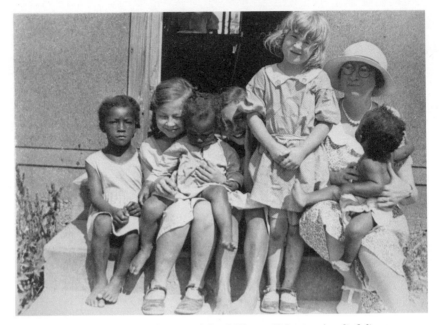

*Louise Armstrong poses with some of the children of Manistee's relief clients.*
(Louise Armstrong collection, Bentley Historical Library, University of Michigan)

changed from county to county and city to city. Despite the government's claims, the scientific precision of federal food relief was illusory. Instead, the diet fed to millions of Americans was experimental, based on a new science and shaped by such unknowns as the inclinations of the administrator, the politics of local officials, and the state of the local economy. In Manistee, a county that had been in depression since the turn of the century, food allowances were only slightly higher than they had been during the days of the poor commission.

The two controllable variables were the type and amount of food that clients were allowed to receive. Michigan's relief distributions used a card or voucher system. In place of cash, the client was given a pink-colored form, in duplicate, with two printed columns running down the length of the paper. The column was broken up by headings such as Meats, Cereals, Canned Goods, and

Vegetables. Under each heading, the relief agency specified the particular items allowed that week and what they could total. The grocer held on to the top form so he could be reimbursed, while the duplicate was sent to the relief office to verify client compliance. There was something about the intrusiveness of those pink food vouchers, so easy to spot by fellow shoppers. As one relief client explained:

> *The food ticket is an instrument that puts your soul in limbo while leaving your body among the free. I can still hardly believe we ever accepted the degrading thing. But I know we did. Once you've accepted the hospitality of the nation the steps downward seem to be greased. I wonder at what point of his descent it appears natural to a man to pick up a cigar stump from the gutter.*[3]

For many people on relief, the image of that stooped figure at the curb, so much at odds with the myth of American self-sufficiency, was an accurate representation of what charity could do to a person. The shame of accepting it was not so much imposed as internalized, bubbling up freely from within.

While Hopkins insisted on the nutritional soundness of the FERA diet, those actually on the relief rolls felt differently. In fact, the meagerness of government rations unleashed a wave of protests against state relief administrations. In New York, Los Angeles, Dallas, Oklahoma City, Wichita, and many other cities, demonstrators besieged emergency relief offices. The authorities dismissed them as left-wing troublemakers, but it was harder to ignore the criticisms of more disinterested observers. In early 1934, Helen Hart, a supervisor with Connecticut's Emergency Relief Commission, suggested that local church families, as a spiritual exercise, try living on a relief diet for a week during Lent to "share the experiences of thousands of their fellow citizens." Twenty-five families signed up for the weeklong experiment. Seventeen families were given grocery orders based on the standards for an "Adequate Diet at Minimum Cost." Three single women based their meals on the $2.50-a-week budget suggested by the state, and five families received food directly from Hartford's Municipal Commissary. After just a week of the experimental diet, test subjects had already begun to feel its effects. One minister lost two pounds on the "adequate" regimen; his wife lost three, as did the maid and the two older children. The baby remained the same weight, but only because his mother had given him part of her rations. Families fed by the Municipal Commissary found that by the end of the week their children had become noticeably irritable. Adults were unhappy as well. When they demanded some kind of seasoning for their food, welfare supervisors refused. A relief family granted vinegar and mustard, they reasoned, might "begin to feel too much like other families" and lose the will to support themselves.

When news broke about the Hartford experiment, Hopkins offered no defense. Instead, he welcomed the publicity as repudiation of the "prevailing impression that food budgets were unnecessarily liberal." In 1934, as the national economy began to pick up, Hopkins increased food relief budgets, but only slightly. Haunted by the fear of giving too much and inviting dependence, he preferred to address deficiencies in the relief diet through education. To help clients make better use of what they already had, each relief office was encouraged to hire its own resident home economist. In concert with schools, churches, and settlement houses, home economists employed by FERA distributed fact sheets and recipes and arranged for cooking and nutrition classes. For more personalized instruction, they trained a corps of unemployed women to serve as visiting housekeepers who went from home to home teaching women how to select "nutritious and palatable foods" and prepare them in "simple and appetizing combinations."[4] Government cooking classes were well attended. In one of the poorest sections of Chicago, six hundred mothers sat through a nutrition demonstration in their children's school, learning how to cook three meals a day at eighteen cents per person. In New York City public schools, women who "in normal times could not be induced to enroll in such classes" signed up by the thousands for government cooking lessons. As a result of the Depression, even experienced home cooks felt unprepared:

> *Keeping the family nourished on half of what we had to spend four years ago takes more than womanly instinct and maternal advice. It takes knowing whether you get more protein for your money in eggs or meat, whether there's enough calcium for Johnny's bones and teeth in spinach or do you have to buy the more expensive vegetables. It takes knowledge of the chemistry of cooking: the effects of heat on vitamins, and how to cook cheap cuts of meat so that they are nourishing and palatable.*[5]

Women wanted food knowledge, and the government was on hand to provide it.

———

AT THE SAME time that millions were going hungry, American farmers were letting crops go unharvested. During the 1920s, the postwar collapse of agricultural prices had driven farmers to produce record crops just to stay afloat. By the 1930s, prices had fallen so prohibitively low that the cost of harvesting crops and transporting them to market was more than many farmers could afford. Instead, like the California farmers in Steinbeck's *Grapes of Wrath*, they left food to rot in the fields:

> *And the first cherries ripen. Cent and a half a pound. Hell, we can't pick 'em for that. Black and red cherries, full and sweet, and the birds eat half of each cherry and the yellowjackets buzz*

*into the holes the birds made. . . . The purple prunes soften and*
*sweeten. My God, we can't pick them and dry them and sulfur*
*them. We can't pay wages, no matter what the wages.*[6]

But the "saddest, bitterest thing of all" was the purposeful destruction of wholesome food. In California, citrus growers sprayed carloads of oranges with kerosene to deter foragers, while in Wisconsin dairymen protesting federal farm policy dumped 40,000 pounds of milk onto the highway. For people living through the Depression, stories about food that had been dumped from trucks or thrown into ditches were impossible to reconcile with images of breadlines and news about the rising incidence of childhood malnutrition. By 1932, "the paradox of want amid plenty," a phrase coined by the journalist Walter Lippmann, had become a theme of the Great Depression. Under Roosevelt, attempts to resolve it led to a series of government interventions that would bring food to millions of relief families.

Pressed by farm state politicians to end surpluses and stabilize falling prices, in May 1933, President Roosevelt created the Agricultural Adjustment Administration. The AAA's first move was to plow under nearly a quarter of the nation's cotton fields. To stem a glut in the hog market, it next arranged to slaughter millions of young pigs and pregnant sows, their carcasses left to decompose in Chicago rail yards or dumped into the Mississippi. As news of the waste spread, Americans grew outraged. With typical alacrity, Roosevelt shifted course and created the Federal Surplus Relief Corporation to buy up surplus food and distribute it to the unemployed. Led by Harry Hopkins, the corporation undertook its first job: the distribution of twenty-three million pounds of pork.

In October 1933, Louise Armstrong received orders to send a truck to the next county to pick up Manistee's share of federal salt pork. The meat was then divided into six-pound parcels and delivered to relief clients by a volunteer driver in a borrowed truck. The driver, who had lived in Manistee all his life, was shocked by the living conditions he encountered:

> *Folks with a bunch of kids, and old folks—living in shanties that ain't fit for pigs—sometimes without even no floor, only dirt. I had a hard time making some of 'em understand about the pork. Some thought I was trying to sell it to 'em, and when I said not, they wanted to know if it was really for them, and finally I sez it was a present from the Government. A lot of 'em—especially the old folks—broke down and cried. I guess all some of 'em had to eat is potatoes and beans and bread, and not too much of any of that. Some said they hadn't tasted meat for months.*[7]

Salt pork was just the first of many foods to flow through the surplus commodities pipeline. Between 1933 and 1935, FERA sent millions of tons of "government food" for distribution in every state of the union. Over two years, Michigan alone received fifteen million pounds of pork, seven million pounds of canned beef, and train cars filled with flour, butter, potatoes, eggs, lard, wheat, breakfast cereal, beans, cheese, and fresh beef and veal. Without a precedent to follow, Armstrong had to cobble together a system for storing and distributing government food. Her first necessity was for cold storage, which she found in an empty storefront on Main Street. In the summer of 1934, yet another massive drought hit the Great Plains from North Dakota down to Texas. As it wore on, and cattle began to suffer, the government purchased more than six million head of half-starved cattle and sheep and sent them to slaughter. Much of the meat was canned, but some of the carcasses were chilled and sent to any county that could process them. With its cold storage facility, one of those counties was Manistee. For Armstrong's clients the five-pound packages of fresh beef and veal were a godsend.

Government dry goods were initially stored at the FERA office.

When it began to overflow, Armstrong rented a warehouse, which she put under the supervision of a relief client named Henry. For two years, Henry (and his cat) kept the government warehouse neat, clean, and free of mice. As the old frame building filled with supplies, it became a symbol of hope for Armstrong, who took pleasure in gazing over its well-ordered contents:

> *On the way home, we stop at the warehouse. Henry is anxious to have me see the bins the men have been building to take care of the garden products. . . . The big one for the potatoes extends almost the full length of the building, and is already partly filled. I think of our school children from relief families eating those good baked potatoes this winter, with lots of good government butter on them. Perhaps by spring some of those little faces will not look so pinched.*[8]

Armstrong recruited grocery stores to act as distribution centers, identified by signs hung in their windows: GOVERNMENT FOOD ORDERS FILLED HERE! The system ran smoothly for a time, but store owners eventually began to grumble about so many nonpaying customers. Rumors began to circulate about renegade grocers demanding money from FERA clients and tainting FERA food. Armstrong responded by cutting out the grocers and setting up a commissary for dispensing food. For families living out in the countryside, she arranged for a truck delivery system. Twice a month bundles of food were packed and transported to a post office or school or country store where clients could collect their supplies. In summer they arrived with wagons to help carry the food home, and in winter, sleds.

In Washington, the Bureau of Home Economics seized on federal food distributions as another educational opportunity. In the fall of 1933, government salt pork entered American kitchens with instructions attached, courtesy of the bureau: "Salt pork is an all around meat. You can serve it fried, with milk and gravy; or with cereals and vegetables in 1-dish meals; or in sandwiches and many other savory ways." Among the recipes that followed were fried salt pork with biscuits and gravy ("a good supper menu for a cold winter evening"), salt pork and scalloped vegetables, baked salt pork, salt pork stew, salt pork scrapple, and salt pork sandwiches in which the cooked meat was mixed with any combination of chopped eggs, raw cabbage, cottage cheese, and pickles.[9] As FERA prepared to distribute five million pounds of beans, Aunt Sammy took to the airwaves briefing homemakers on legume nutrition. A government distribution of canned meat in the winter of 1934 was her cue for a lesson on canned meat cookery. The key to success, she explained, was to reverse the normal cooking order and add the meat *last*, as in this recipe for meat-and-turnip pie devised by the Bureau of Home Economics and distributed by FERA in the winter of 1934:

———•◦•———

Cook 1 quart diced turnips tender in 1 quart boiled salted water. Thicken with flour mixed with cold water. Add one pint cut-up canned meat, and pour into a shallow pan or baking dish. Cover with dough and bake in a hot oven. For this dough sift 1 quart of flour with 1½ teaspoons salt and 2 tablespoons baking powder. Work in 4 tablespoons of fat. Add enough liquid (water, or fresh milk or dried or evaporated milk made up with water) about 1½ cups to make a soft dough. Roll out and pat the dough about ¾ inch thick. Cover the pie with the sheet of dough or cut it into biscuits and place them close together over the top of the meat-and-turnip mixture.[10]

———•◦•———

To facilitate milk distribution, FERA made it available in a number of forms—fresh, evaporated, condensed, and powdered.

In 1934, it added yet another product to the dairy lineup, this one engineered by Flora Rose. Back in the 1920s, Columbia nutritionist Henry Sherman had discovered that rats fed a diet of two-thirds ground wheat and one-third dry skim milk saw a 10 percent increase in their life span. Making the leap from rodents to hominids, he extrapolated that humans fed the same food would show comparable health benefits. In 1932, with increasing numbers of Americans threatened by malnutrition, Flora Rose decided it was time to produce Sherman's wonder food and developed a line of breakfast cereals inspired by his formula. Milkorno, Milkwheato, and Milkoato were three of America's first fortified foods. With great fanfare, Rose introduced Milkorno, the first of the cereals, at Cornell's February 1933 Farm & Home Week, where the assembled dignitaries—including Eleanor Roosevelt, wife of the president-elect—were fed a budget meal that included a Milkorno polenta with tomato sauce. The price tag per person was 6½ cents. FERA chose Milkwheato (manufactured under the Cornell Research Foundation's patent) to add to its shipments of surplus foods, contracting with the Grange League Federation and the Ralston Purina Company to manufacture it. In early 1934, four pounds of Milkwheato were added to the monthly rations of millions of families. In Michigan, Lelia McGuire, the state's nutrition director, considered Milkwheato an essential part of the "minimal" relief diet, reminding her staff that a diet of whole wheat and skimmed milk had sustained rats through more than thirty generations![11]

Milkwheato and its sister cereals represented the pinnacle of scientifically enlightened eating. Forerunners to our own protein bars and nutritional shakes, they were high in nutrients, inexpensive, and nonperishable. White in color and with no pronounced flavor of their own, they were versatile too. Easily adapted to a variety of culinary applications, they boosted the nutritional value of whatever dish they touched. They could be baked into muffins, cookies, biscuits, and breads; stirred into chowders and chili con carne;

mixed into meat loaf; and even used in place of noodles in Chinese chop suey. Here is a version of that Chinese-American classic, as interpreted by Cornell's Department of Home Economics:

CHOP SUEY WITH MILKORNO

2 pounds lean pork cut in cubes
2 cups sliced celery
2 cups sliced onions
salt and pepper to taste
3 or 4 cups cooked milkorno

Saute pork; add the seasonings and ½ cup water and simmer until tender. About ½ hour before meat is tender add the celery and onions. If desired the gravy may be thickened by adding 2 tablespoons of flour to each cup of liquid. Pour this mixture over hot cooked milkorno, and serve.[12]

DURING THE GREAT War, America had discovered the strategic value of morale, that "go get 'em" spirit that would carry the Allies to victory. Both on and off the battlefield, boosting morale became the work of popular songs, movies, government posters, newsreels, comic strips, and bond rallies. Newspapers ran editorials on the importance of morale and monitored its fluctuations. During the Depression, concerns about morale resurfaced, only this time, in place of the troops, their object was "the standing army of the unemployed." Applied to a new kind of conflict, "morale" during the Depression was mainly defined by its absence. Most crucially, as a man lost morale he also lost the desire to work.

As America's "minister of relief," Harry Hopkins was afraid

that government charity could wind up destroying the work ethic of an entire generation. However, he was fully behind any kind of government supported self-help program that allowed people to produce their own food. The subsistence gardens bank-rolled by FERA had their origins in the Hoover administration. As a son of rural Iowa, Hoover saw the family farm as the ideal expression of American self-sufficiency. Roosevelt, a gentleman farmer raised on his family's Hyde Park estate, also had a life-long bias toward the superior economic and moral worth of farm life and as governor had urged the unemployed to leave the tenements for clean air and clean living in the countryside. Under his direction, TERA brought vegetable gardens to towns and cities throughout the state, including 2,400 tilled acres in New York City alone. Like his boss, Hopkins believed that giving a jobless man a rake and hoe would "lift him out of the mental state into which idleness inevitably plunges him," and as director of federal relief, he expanded community and subsistence gardening across the nation.[13]

In Manistee, with seeds provided by the government, community gardens produced carrots, turnips, squash, and nearly two thousand bushels of potatoes, all distributed to the poor. Out in the countryside, clients were given free seeds to till their own plots, called thrift gardens. (In many states, relief administrators denied food orders to any able-bodied client who refused to plant a garden.) To make the most of the harvest, in thousands of counties around the nation, FERA set up community canning stations, allowing "thrift gardeners" the use of equipment they could not otherwise afford. In bigger towns, canning stations were set up in municipal buildings and furnished with steam-heated pressure cookers and sealing machines. In poor sections of the rural South, farmers built tin-roofed canning centers with screen windows, though most of the canning process took place outdoors on stoves made out of gasoline drums. All canning stations were staffed with an instructor familiar with the latest and safest canning methods, as prescribed by the Bureau of Home Economics. In one remote Oregon county, an instructor traveled from farm to farm on a mobile cannery made from an old truck and some discarded factory equipment. Demand for instruction was so strong that the truck was kept busy day and night.

In 1934, Michigan's unemployed tilled 85,000 thrift gardens, while the state's canning centers preserved roughly two million quarts of vegetables. In home kitchens, women with more food than the family could use preserved it and gave it away in charity canning drives like the one organized by the American Legion in Benton Harbor, Michigan. "If you are going to make jellies and jams this summer," ran a story in the local paper, "why not follow the example of the many unselfish women who are putting up a few gift glasses every time they make a batch of jelly for their own families?" The following is a recipe for paradise jelly, a garnet-colored preserve made from quince, crabapple, and cranberry, three fruits harvested late in the season:

<hr>

## PARADISE JELLY

Twenty crabapples
10 quinces
1 quart cranberries

Wash and pick over cranberries. Wash crabapples and
quinces and cut into small pieces, cutting out blossom
end and all defective parts. Put into kettle with enough
cold water to cover and add cranberries. Cover and cook
until soft. Strain through jelly bag. Measure juice. Bring
to the boiling point and for every cup of juice add one cup
sugar. Boil, skimming as necessary, and when syrup sheets

from spoon turn into sterilized jelly glasses and cover with paraffin. Cover with a second layer of paraffin when cold. It will take about eight minutes to cook the juice and sugar.[14]

---

LATE IN 1934, a field investigator named Edward Webster handed in a report to his boss, Harry Hopkins, that seemed to bear out the FERA director's darkest predictions. In Missouri, Oklahoma, Arkansas, and Texas, Webster found that the unemployed had stopped bothering to look for work and were now heading directly to the relief office. As a result, relief loads were inexorably rising. Once a relief client was on board, the report continued, his values and attitudes underwent "radical modification." People who had once shuddered at the idea of charity lapsed into a comfortable state of dependency, and before too long were demanding relief as "one of the rights of American citizens."[15] Federal relief was never meant for the long haul. Webster's report, one in a series of similar sentiment, only hastened the inevitable.

In a historic first, President Roosevelt's 1935 state of the union address was both broadcast on radio *and* recorded on film. With the House of Representatives ablaze with klieg lights and a raucous audience overflowing the galleries into the aisles and down the corridors, the occasion might have been mistaken for a Hollywood premiere. The mood changed, however, when an unsmiling Roosevelt began to speak. To anyone who had taken heart at his inauguration promises, his announcement that day seemed to emanate from a different man. Both history and recent experience, the president said,

> *show conclusively that continued dependence upon relief induces a spiritual and moral disintegration fundamentally destructive to the national fiber. To dole out relief in this way is to administer a narcotic, a subtle destroyer of the human spirit. It*

*is inimical to the dictates of sound policy. It is in violation of the traditions of America.*[16]

While the job of giving relief would go back to counties and local politicians, the federal government would embark on a vast new program that came to be known as the Works Progress Administration. Armstrong says repeatedly that her book is just *an account of her experiences,* not a defense or critique of one relief policy over another. But she can't hold back, and gives her opinion anyway. In her telling, when control was returned to the counties, the whole relief system was recontaminated by the crooks and power brokers who had run it for years. When Armstrong saw the hopelessness of the situation, she resigned. For two years, federal relief had been "a fearless, honest effort to relieve human suffering," but that period was over, and another was starting.

# Chapter 8

———•◦•———

**T**WO WEEKS INTO his new administration, in a show of
gastronomic solidarity with the American people, President Roosevelt sat down to a modest lunch of hot deviled
eggs in tomato sauce, mashed potatoes, and, for dessert, prune
pudding. In what would become a daily routine, lunch that day
had been rolled into the Oval Office to be eaten at the president's
desk. Here, just twenty-four hours earlier, FDR had signed a bill
to reduce federal spending by cutting veterans' benefits. The economy menu was part of a new austerity program adopted by the
White House to show America that the first family, too, was cutting costs. No sacrifice had been made, however, when it came to
nutrition. On the contrary, the president's budget lunch provided
a balanced composition of calories and nutrients: eggs for iron and
protein, potatoes for energy, prunes and tomatoes for vitamins A
and C. And all for a total of 7½ cents! When reporters asked the
president what he thought of the food, he answered that it was
"good" and that he had cleaned his plate. For any homemaker inspired to cook the same meal for her own family, the newspapers
included recipes for all three dishes. Prune pudding, a molded
dessert thickened by a slurry of flour and water, was one of many
Depression-era dishes to make use of dried fruit, the more economical alternative to fresh:

## PRUNE PUDDING

One-fourth pound prunes, one-half cupful cold water, one-half cupful sugar, two cupfuls prune water, one inch stick of cinnamon, one-fourth teaspoonful powdered cinnamon, four tablespoonsful of flour, four tablespoonsful cold water.

Soak prunes overnight in one and one-half cupfuls cold water. Cook in same water until tender over slow fire in covered dish. Drain. Save liquid. Remove seeds, cut prunes into bits. Add sugar, cinnamon and hot prune juice—if juice does not measure two cupfuls add enough water to make up the measure.

Bring to boiling point and simmer ten minutes. To the flour add four tablespoonfuls of cold water and mix to a smooth paste. Add slowly to the prune mixture, stirring carefully and cook for ten minutes over a low fire or over boiling water. Remove stick of cinnamon and pour into a bowl or mold. Serve cold.[1]

Food, like language, is always in motion, propelled by the same events that fill our history books. Wars, advances in science and technology, and shifting patterns of migration and commerce are continuously shaping and reshaping the foods that sustain us. During the 1930s, home economists took it upon themselves to interrupt a typically organic process and, in one colossal push, replace traditional foodways with a scientifically designed eating program. With roots stretching all the way back to the mid-nineteenth century, their vision was not exactly new. The Depression, however, had galvanized an already committed group of reformers, their renewed determination matched by growing fears of malnutrition felt by ordinary Americans. But if the country was finally ready for change, nothing could happen without nutritional standards. The job of creating them was taken up by a female-dominated branch of the United States Department of Agriculture called the Bureau of Home Economics.

The bureau's founding was the culmination of a four-decade-long relationship between home economists and the federal government. As far back as Wilbur O. Atwater and his calorimeter, home economists had been on the scene, working as laboratory assistants for the eminent scientist. What they learned from Atwater, they applied to practical kitchen tasks, the results of their studies published by the USDA. (One of the earliest, *Bread and the Principles of Bread Making,* was by Atwater's daughter, Helen, who would go on to become the editor of the *Journal of Home Economics.*) In 1907, the government's nutrition studies were moved from Connecticut, Atwater's home base, into the Washington offices of the USDA. Here, a small room was set up as a kitchen laboratory that eventually became the hub of the Office of Home Economics, which was established in 1915.

During World War I, the government kitchen became a hotbed of culinary research. With food conservation a matter of national security, home economists dropped whatever food projects they were working on to figure out what Americans should eat now that beef, pork, wheat, and sugar were being shipped overseas to feed the troops and were temporarily off the home-front menu. Using Atwater's substitution theory, they developed an emergency diet that used cornmeal and barley flour in place of wheat, honey and sorghum instead of sugar, and beans and nuts rather than animal protein. Conservation recipes were formulated, printed up as cards, and distributed to homemakers around the country. Recipes, though, took home cooks only as far as the next meal. To plan menus, women also needed to understand the science behind the recipes. Food guides published during the war, like Lucy Gillett's

*Food Primer for the Home,* filled that role, introducing women to vitamins, calories, and the concept of food groups, knowledge they could use to plan balanced menus long after the war was over.

Having proved its usefulness in a national emergency, the Office of Home Economics was promoted to the status of bureau in 1923. There was no corresponding raise, however, in government funds. The new bureau was housed in the temporary dormitories built for women defense workers during the war and had just seven employees. Louise Stanley, the bureau chief, was a forty-year-old professor of home economics from rural Tennessee who had earned a doctorate in chemistry at Yale. Over the next twenty years, Stanley would stake out a place for home economics in the federal government, gathering under one roof the largest staff of female scientists

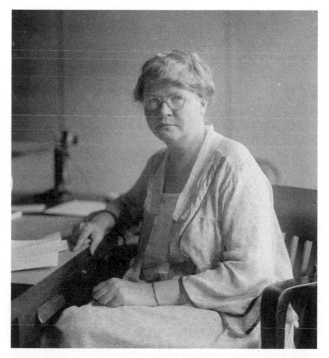

*Louise Stanley, chief of the Bureau of Home Economics from 1923 to 1943.* (National Photo Company Collection, Library of Congress, LC-DIG-npcc-24560)

anywhere in the country. The bureau was organized into three fact-finding divisions: Clothing and Textiles, Economics, and Food and Nutrition. The research objective of all three was to develop a body of best housekeeping practices, scientifically tested protocols and procedures that women could refer to for expert instruction. What that meant in terms of food was setting dietary standards, quantitative guidelines for feeding the family, similar to Atwater's, only updated to include the newer vitamin research. But arriving at those numbers—the holy grail of American nutritionists—would take years of investigation. In the meantime, women had everyday food problems to be solved, which the bureau treated with the utmost in scientific rigor. Bureau scientists tackled questions like which cooking fat delivered the flakiest piecrust, what was the ideal storage temperature for sweet potatoes, and how to prepare a tender Sunday roast—a study that ran a full six years. When sufficient information was gathered, it was written up as a government bulletin and sent out to any woman who requested a copy.

Every year the bureau received a regular stream of letters requesting professional help on some aspect of cleaning, cooking, or sewing. In 1931, letters began pouring in from women struggling to feed their children. Many of the women who worked at the bureau, Stanley included, had been active in the food education drive launched during the war. With past experience a dress rehearsal for the current emergency, in 1931 the bureau began a campaign to flood the American public with information on food and nutrition. For the most current research, they looked to Henry Sherman at Columbia University and Elmer V. McCollum of vitamin fame. Before the science could be disseminated, however, the bureau had to sift it, strip it down, and translate it into concrete food recommendations. In 1930, Hazel Stiebeling, the bureau's newly hired food economist, had cobbled together an emergency diet for people affected by the southern drought. The following year, those mimeographed pages were refined and expanded into a little booklet called *Adequate Diets for People of Limited Income*, the first in a series of increasingly sophisticated federal food guides.

An Ohio farm girl, Stiebeling had as a college student discovered Henry Sherman's *The Chemistry of Food and Nutrition* and was immediately captivated, plowing through half the book at the first sitting. Stiebeling attended Columbia University, where she worked under Sherman, receiving her doctorate in chemistry in 1928. Two years later, she joined the bureau as a senior food economist. The food guides issued by the bureau served both as prescriptions for rational eating and nutritional primers. They familiarized readers with each of the known vitamins and minerals and described their contribution to maintaining good health, information that for most people was sketchy at best.

During the war, home economists like Lucy Gillett had been confident that with expert guidance even the poor could afford good nutrition. Depression-era food guides accepted the much bleaker reality that some Americans were insufficiently fed—even in times of prosperity—and were now so poor that a balanced diet was beyond their means. The worst off were southern sharecroppers, who according to the bureau were not only vitamin starved but also averse to a healthy variety of foods. In deference to culinary custom, the bureau advised a suitably limited diet that left poor southerners open to pellagra, a glaring instance of racial bias masquerading as cultural sensitivity.[2] Published in 1933, *Diets at Four Levels of Nutritive Content and Cost* was Stiebeling's technical treatise on eating according to income bracket, followed three years later by *Diets to Fit the Family Income*, a layperson's guide based on the same formula.

The first step for readers of *Diets to Fit the Family Income* was to find their place on Stiebeling's income scale. Those at the high end, households earning more than $5,000 ($85,000 today) a year, were granted a "Liberal Diet" of varied foods in generous amounts. A "Moderate Diet," which contained fewer of the protective foods but which Stiebeling assured readers was still "fully satisfactory in all nutritional details," was for families in the $3,000 to $4,000 bracket. A "Minimum Diet," designed for households earning between $1,000 and $2,000, met all nutritional needs, but as cheaply as possible, with just enough fruits and vegetables, eggs, and meat to maintain overall health.[3] Where resources were extremely meager, however, the family's sole option was a "Restricted Diet," recommended only for short periods. Based on bread and milk, the "Restricted Diet" provided no margin of safety in the case of unforeseen calamities like a scorched pot of beans or moldy bag of flour. A selection of menus showing how each of the four diets might translate into actual meals gave solidity to the culinary differences between rich and poor, a particularly bitter illustration for those in the bottom tiers, the women most likely to need such a publication.

---

NUTRITION IN THE 1930s was an emotionally fraught topic. Vitamins, both invisible and fragile, were especially concerning. More than anything else, women were afraid of the "hidden hunger" caused by undetectable vitamin deficiencies that could well be injuring their children. In a letter to Louise Stanley, Lucy Gillett observed that the Depression seemed "to have crystallized a nutrition consciousness throughout the country," with more people "inquiring how they might protect the health of their children than ever before." Home economists leveraged those fears. To ensure compliance, bureau food guides came with stark admonitions, warning mothers that poor nutrition in childhood could handicap a person for life. Women were left with the impression that one false move on their part meant their children would grow up with night blindness and bowed knees.

Aunt Sammy, on the other hand, on the radio show *Housekeepers' Chat* made it all sound manageable. As the Depression progressed, Aunt Sammy became the bureau's voice of reassurance, assuaging the country's nutritional fears in her small-town cadence. On the subject of vitamins, she had this to say: "Most of us who have a simple but varied diet, and are without food prejudices, get our supply of vitamins whether we think about it or not."[4] Her taste in food was equally no-nonsense. Aunt Sammy appreciated the frugal standbys that were a regular part of America's ancestral diet but that had more recently fallen out of favor. Cracked whole wheat, an ingredient traditionally used to make breakfast porridge, was one of the old-time economy foods promoted by bureau nutritionists. Aunt Sammy became its champion. Here she is in a 1932 broadcast elaborating on the virtues of this generally unfamiliar food, an item that many of her listeners would have associated with animal feed:

> *Maybe it's my Scotch blood. Maybe it's the early training from a thrifty grandmother. Maybe it's the hungry people I've seen and the undernourished children. Anyway, I always hate to see good food going to waste, especially when pocketbooks are thin. That's why I want to remind you today about one of our best foods which has been neglected by housewives in recent years. Whole wheat, wheat in the kernel, is plentiful and cheap these days especially in the wheat belt. You can get wheat at the feed store or mill or maybe from a farmer in your neighborhood. Yet, many people I've been hearing about have gone hungry because they don't know how to use this wheat, how to fix it in tasteful dishes that the whole family will enjoy.[5]*

Whole wheat in milk chowder with carrots, onions, parsley, and pork; whole wheat with diced beef and chili pepper; whole wheat scalloped with liver and bacon; and whole wheat stewed with tomatoes and served on toast were a few of Aunt Sammy's cooking suggestions. Another concoction—whole wheat, fish, and tomatoes—exemplifies the bureau's continuing effort to find new applications for low-cost ingredients:

————

## WHOLE WHEAT, FISH AND TOMATOES

½ pound canned fish

1 quart canned tomatoes

½ cup chopped celery

½ teaspoon pepper

2 cups cooked whole wheat

Drain the fish, reserve the liquid and flake the fish into small pieces. Cook tomatoes, celery and fish liquid until the mixture is fairly thick. Add the seasoning, wheat, and fish, cook a few minutes longer, stir to blend well.[6]

————

Well aware that its Depression diet was based on foods that many people would have preferred not to eat, the bureau was always looking for ways to counteract food biases. One strategy was to dress up low-status foods like beans, a critical source of cheap protein. To impart a touch of elegance to a bowl of split pea soup, why not float a thin slice of lemon on top and sprinkle it with some bright red paprika and finely chopped parsley? Or beans could be mashed, formed into dainty patties, and fried like croquettes. Here, for a novel bean presentation, Aunt Sammy suggests using them as a stuffing:

————

## STUFFED ONIONS

Cut large onions in half, simmer in lightly salted water until almost tender. Lift the onions out and remove the center rings, chop and mix with cooked or canned beans. Season to taste with salt and pepper and fill the onion shells with the mixture. Sprinkle bread crumbs on top and bake in the oven until the onions are tender and brown on top.[7]

The bureau's Information Service was prolific and well coordinated. The release of each new food guide and recipe circular was synchronized both with Aunt Sammy's *Housekeepers' Chat* and with a weekly newspaper food column called *The Market Basket* created by the bureau in 1931. The same information was carried into rural America by home extension agents, government-paid instructors connected with the country's land grant colleges, who used the bureau's food guides as their textbooks.

In 1934, the bureau attracted the attention of a media ally, a writer who not only helped spread the bureau's message but also adopted it as his personal credo. In the 1920s, Gove Hambidge had become interested in the marriage between modern science and food production and published a series of articles in *Ladies' Home Journal* about how that union was changing the national cuisine. With help from bacteriologists, chemists, and engineers, he reported, food manufacturers were supplying the public with products of unparalleled purity and consistency. In home kitchens, women were reaping the benefits of science in the forms of labor-saving devices and canned or "frosted" foods that defied the old laws of seasonal availability. The "New Era in Food," however, was interrupted by the Depression. Moved by the economic crisis, Hambidge turned his focus from food technology to nutrition, another facet of the scientific revolution that was reshaping American foodways. The Bureau of Home Economics could not have asked for a more dedicated spokesperson. Published in

*Ladies' Home Journal*, his article "Make the Diet Fit the Pocket-book," an explanation of Stiebeling's four diets for four income levels, reached more than two and a half million readers. Over the next year, he expanded the article into *Your Meals and Your Money*, a book-length explication of Stiebeling's principles written for a mass audience. The following year, Hambidge quit the magazine business and got a job with the United States Department of Agriculture, where he continued to advocate for nutrition education.

INFORMATION FROM THE BUREAU flowed through many channels. Its patron, however, was Eleanor Roosevelt. Before the Roosevelts had even moved into the White House, Eleanor wrote to Louise Stanley suggesting the two women meet, part of her plan to convene Washington's "women executives" and harness their combined talents. Over the next decade, the two women carried on a regular correspondence, with Stanley a frequent guest at the first lady's all-women press conferences. In her personal appearances, in print, and on the radio, Eleanor kept the public informed about the bureau's work. Early that first spring, as a guest on a USDA radio show called the *National Farm and Home Hour*, she endorsed the bureau's diet for children, stressing the importance of feeding one's child the "right proportions" as outlined by government scientists. In these hard times, food is vital to our children's health, she told the nation, "and not merely any food you happen to have, but the right kind of food."[8] From time to time, the bureau was attacked as an example of government bureaucracy run amok. When conservative critics asked why government money should pay for research on how to clean rugs and put up preserves, Eleanor dashed off a letter to the newspapers. The countless people helped by the bureau, she insisted, had more than compensated for its small cost to American taxpayers.[9] As the bureau well knew, Eleanor's stamp of approval was a public relations windfall. A few words from the first lady on any subject and it "takes on an importance it could acquire in no other way" was how the bureau's information chief described Eleanor's influence, second only to that of the president himself.[10]

In a more personal act of patronage, Eleanor brought home economics into the White House. On a visit to Cornell early in 1933, Eleanor sampled one of the economy meals devised by her friend Flora Rose. On the menu that day was polenta made with Milkorno, the nutritional compound developed by Rose to feed the unemployed. Eleanor was favorably impressed—in fact, so much so that she decided to continue the diet at home. Events like this, staged tastings in which people of note—politicians mostly—publicly endorsed Depression menus, had become a kind of civic ritual. No politician, however, was expected to extend the sacrifice and make these economy meals a regular habit. That was partly because most of the tasters were men. Eleanor, however, on the verge of becoming first lady and running the country's most scrutinized household, saw a teaching opportunity. She already believed that home economics could deliver women from the drudgery of traditional housekeeping. The budget lunch demonstrated what those same women could contribute to society in a time of crisis. The woman who practiced balanced nutrition guarded her family's health—and by extension that of the country—when it was most at risk. Born to a household full of servants, Eleanor had little firsthand kitchen experience. By her own account, the one dish she cooked for the family was scrambled eggs, prepared *à table* in a large silver chafing dish. An unlikely gastronomic role model, as first lady Eleanor nonetheless was in a unique position to showcase the food recommended by home economists and inspire America's home cooks. And what better way to make her point than by serving the same food to her own family?

The president's budget luncheon signaled a culinary regime change at the White House. Going forward, the first family would eat turkey tetrazzini and corned beef hash, just like normal

Americans. At Eleanor's decree, culinary economizing was extended to guests as well, a directive she put into action on her first day in the White House. The inaugural lunch menu consisted of cold jellied bouillon, chicken and salmon salads, and bread and butter sandwiches—a long way from the elaborate spreads that had been par for the course at such gala occasions. For dinner that night, she requested oyster stew with crackers, scrambled eggs, creamed chicken, peas, rolls, and biscuits, "a New England countryman's supper," as the White House butler described it.[11] Staff members familiar with how things were done in the White House were scandalized by the departure from culinary precedent. However, Eleanor also had her allies. The new housekeeper, fifty-nine-year-old Henrietta Nesbitt, whom the first lady had brought down from Hyde Park, shared her employer's appreciation for "plain food, plainly cooked." A homemaker with no professional kitchen experience, Nesbitt was in charge of all provisioning and menu planning, her culinary fingerprints easily recognized in dishes like ham loaf and chipped beef and noodle casserole, foods more at home in a school lunchroom than the presidential mansion.

Under Nesbitt's supervision, the White House put out not only some of the dreariest food in Washington but also some of the most dismally prepared. Though Nesbitt was not personally behind the stove, "she stood over the cooks, making sure that each dish was overcooked or undercooked or ruined one way or another."[12] Dinner guests, appalled by the consistently miserable cooking they encountered at the White House table, recorded their gastronomic misadventures. Senator Hiram Johnson described a meal with FDR that included "indifferent chowder," followed by "some mutton served in slices already cut which had become almost cold, with peas that were none too palatable."[13] When Ernest Hemingway was invited to dine at the White House in 1937, he was warned to expect the worst. Still, he was taken aback by the "rainwater soup" and "rubber squab."[14] Lucky

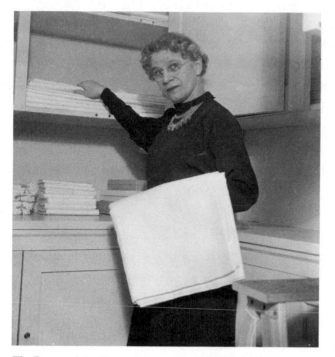

*The Roosevelts' officious housekeeper, Henrietta Nesbitt,*
*1939.* (Harris & Ewing Collection, Library of Congress, LC-DIG-
hec-26752)

for Hemingway, he was spared Mrs. Nesbitt's insipid vegetables, which developed a reputation as one of her many foods to avoid. Experienced invitees came prepared and made sure to eat before leaving the house. Preparedness may also explain the torrent of medical excuses sent in by dinner guests, a strategy of avoidance that Nesbitt picked up on: "Sometimes it seemed to me that practically all the leading men in the world had ulcers, and often when a group of them were having dinner in the White House, we'd have as many as one hundred and fifty forbidden items."[15] Nesbitt was unsympathetic to the "ulcerites," grown men fussing over their food like children.

Her food under attack, she became an expert at deflecting criticism—even when it came from the president. One of FDR's favorite foods was traditionally prepared Maryland terrapin soup. Mrs. Nesbitt's version was watery. When FDR registered his complaint, her feelings were bruised, but only for a little while. She felt much better when she learned that FDR was in a stew over problems with the gold standard, assuring herself that she was the convenient punching bag for his frustrations. This became the pattern. When he complained, she chalked up his grumbling to the pressures of the job and dismissed his comments as more of the same "food peevishness" found in so many other men.[16]

FDR suffered Nesbitt's kitchen tyranny for twelve years, but to be fair, she had been given an impossible assignment. By committing the White House to home economics, Eleanor had volunteered her husband for a culinary experiment that was guaranteed to make him unhappy. FDR recoiled from the plebeian food foisted on him as president; perhaps no dish was more off-putting to him than what home economists referred to as "salads," assemblages made from canned fruit, cream cheese, gelatin, and mayonnaise. A man inclined to indulge his appetites, FDR was partial to fine foods expertly prepared. He was a connoisseur of wild fowl, which he insisted must be eaten rare. He liked his roast beef bloody, too, the juices "pink and running." He enjoyed filet mignon, lobster, oysters, crab, Lake Superior whitefish, and king salmon, boned and planked. He had a special affection for caviar, and pâté de foie gras baked *en croûte*. Eleanor, by contrast, was content with a supper of milk and crackers. "Victuals to her are something to inject into the body" was how her son, James, described his mother's approach to eating.[17] Where other people hankered for a French soufflé, her enjoyment came from non-gustatory sources. "I would be most unhappy if I could not buy new books," she once told a group of women at the White House, "but having beefsteak for dinner would mean nothing to me whatsoever."[18] As first hostess, Eleanor spent countless hours anticipating other people's food desires—her husband's included—but displayed none of her own.

Still, in her way, Eleanor cared about food, not for how it tasted, but for what it *represented*. Scientific cookery, a cuisine of female empowerment, spoke to the feminist in Eleanor. The progressive in her believed that it was good for society. Closer to home, scientific cookery resonated with Eleanor's own ambivalence to the pleasures of the table. Growing up, Eleanor had learned the Protestant virtue of self-denial from her churchgoing mother and grandmother. During the Depression, with millions of Americans destitute, those childhood lessons seemed more pertinent to her than ever before. They helped Eleanor find meaning in the Depression, and as first lady she made it her mission to share them with the rest of the country, the point of her 1933 book, *It's Up to the Women*. Part political manifesto, part homily, and part homemaking manual, *It's Up to the Women* invited American women to break their dependence on material pleasure and return to the values of their more disciplined New England ancestors. To get them started, Eleanor devoted a full chapter to the Cornell diet, the kind of food those abstemious ancestors would have sanctioned. In home economics, Eleanor found a way of thinking about food that was consistent with her values. Built on self-denial, scientific cookery not only dismissed pleasure as nonessential but also treated it as an impediment to healthy eating. Placing too much stock in the way food tasted would steer us to the wrong kinds of foods—rich, highly seasoned, and extravagant. But where our taste buds failed us, science would jump in. Home economists hitched their cause to the most beloved first lady in American history, and with her support they helped reshape the nation's culinary consciousness.

# Chapter 9

————•◦•————

A T THE END of the 1920s, sociologists confidently predicted that the American hobo was a type bound for extinction. Originally migrant workers who hitched rides on the rail lines heading west, hoboes found seasonal jobs laying tracks, following the harvests, and working in the growing country's mines and lumber camps. Observers often confused hoboes with bums, tramps, and other footloose types, but within the subculture differences were clear: "Bums loafs and sits. Tramps loafs and walks. But a hobo moves and works, and he's clean."[1] Generally white, male, native born, and aged between twenty and fifty, hoboes were found across rural America, but they particularly favored the stretch between the Upper Midwest and the Pacific. The glory days of the American hobo lasted from 1870 to 1920. After World War I, most of the rail lines were built; the open frontier was now dotted with towns that could provide their own harvest workers; tractors and combines replaced horse muscle and human sweat; and asphalt roads linked most of the country. The new migrants were families who shuttled from farm to farm in their Ford Model Ts. Once an important part of the country's labor supply, the hobo was in retreat and on the way to obsolescence, a merely picturesque figure in the American landscape.

Before hoboes vanished entirely, however, folklorists and writers infiltrated the migrant world to record their lore, songs, ar-got, and eating habits. From May to November, hoboes generally could be found at work or on the move. In Dakota wheat fields, Oregon lumber camps, and Pacific salmon canneries, employers supplied their workers with simple, filling fare prepared by the camp or mess hall cook. However, hoboes were notoriously restless, often working only a week or two before the itch to travel returned and they hit the trail again. On the road or rails, hoboes' meals were occasionally bought but more often foraged, begged, or stolen. Their emblematic dish was mulligan stew, a descendant of foods served to work gangs on the Union Pacific and other western railways. A properly made "mulligan" was concocted from meat and vegetables begged or stolen from local butchers and grocery stores, the ingredients then stewed in a gallon can over a campfire. When there weren't enough ingredients to make a proper mulligan, the dish became a "slumgullion," or "slum"— the same watery stew that fed the Bonus Army. Farm wives were frequent targets of begging hoboes hoping for a "poke-out," a farmhouse meal wrapped in butcher's paper. This could be "gump" (chicken), "punk and gut" (bread and sausage), "flat cars" (pancakes), "alligator bait" (fried liver), and maybe "jamoke" (coffee) in a paper cup. Sometimes, however, a hobo's luck and ingenuity ran out, leaving him stranded in the middle of nowhere with an empty stomach:

> Oh, my belly is just achin'
> For a couple of strips of bacon,
> A hunk of punk and a little pot of brew.
> I'm tired of the scenery,
> Just lead me to a beanery,
> Where there's something more than air to chew.[2]

In winter when seasonal jobs disappeared, hoboes retreated to the cities, especially Chicago, where the "Main Stem" of West

Madison Street became known as the hobo resort. Here, migrants could find flophouses offering floor space for as little as a nickel a night, saloons, burlesque houses, bordellos, clothing stores selling worn suits and old overcoats, and even a lecture hall called the "Hobo College." For food, they could eat at one of the many workingmen's restaurants serving "Irish turkey" (corned beef and cabbage) or "minister's face" (stewed pig's head) for fifteen cents, hash or liver and onions for a dime, or a sweet roll with coffee for a nickel. The ambience in these cheap eateries was hectic and sanitation nonexistent:

> *The men, a noisy and turbulent crowd, call out their orders, which are shouted by the waiters to the cooks who set out without ceremony the desired dishes. Four or five waiters are able to attend to the wants of a hundred or more men during the course of an hour. The waiters work like madmen during the rush hours, speeding in with orders, out with dirty dishes. During the course of this hour, the waiter becomes literally plastered with splashes of coffee, gravy, and soup. The uncleanliness is revolting and the waiters are no less shocking than the cooks and dishwashers. In the kitchens uncleanliness reaches its limit.*[3]

The bread was usually stale, the hamburger stretched with potatoes and bread crumbs, and the milk sour. Hoboes, however, were in no position to complain and gulped their meals as quickly as possible without looking or smelling. When money ran out, they moved their "flop" to a nearby park for free lodgings and queued up at the mission door for the nightly breadline. This lasted until the leaves returned to the trees and hoboes again felt the stirrings of wanderlust. Then they would visit one of West Madison Street's "slave markets," or employment offices, and sign up to be shipped out on the next train for the great outdoors.

During the 1920s, sociologists watched the yearly influx of migrant workers to Chicago gradually abate as the need for hobo labor shrank. In the autumn of 1930, however, that trend reversed itself as newly jobless men from all walks of life crowded the blocks of West Madison Street. As the first great wave of Depression-era layoffs crested over the city, thousands of men had to figure out new ways to survive. With little government or private charity relief available, following the way of the hobo seemed as good an answer as any. Chicago had relatively few beds in city shelters, so homeless men found accommodation in the area's many hobo camps, or "jungles." Most of these shantytowns were located in vacant lots next to the railroad freight yards. The most famous one was situated right in Grant Park on the downtown waterfront, where homeless men built shacks, some complete with glass windows, stoves, and chimneys, from scavenged wood, tin signs, and other materials. For food, they ate communally, going downtown to round up any ingredients. Back at camp, the "stew-builder," or cook, usually a veteran hobo, would tutor new arrivals on the fine points of preparing a mulligan. In late 1930, the squatters in Grant Park voted to name their community "Hooverville," with thoroughfares dubbed Prosperity Road, Easy Street, and Hard Times Avenue. As the economic crisis became national, Hoovervilles popped up in cities from St. Louis to Seattle to Washington, D.C. "Building may be at a standstill everywhere," said the "mayor" of Chicago's Hooverville, "but down here everything is booming."[4]

From the Hoovervilles and hobo jungles, it was an easy step to hop on one of the freight trains rumbling by and ship out. In the early years of the Great Depression, thousands of Americans hit the roads and rails with little more than a few cents in their pockets. This new "Vagabond Army," driven by a sense of adventure, a need to escape hard times, or, most often, rumors of jobs or more generous relief somewhere over the horizon, was soon discovered by journalists, social workers, photographers, and even movie directors. Between 1932 and 1934, popular magazines ran a spate of articles

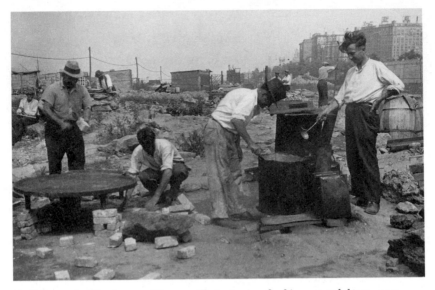

*Residents of a Manhattan Hooverville preparing food in a metal drum, 1932.*
(Authors' collection)

on the new class of wanderers, with special attention given to child hoboes and "lady tramps" often dressed as men. The social dangers of tramp life, where sexual and racial lines were often blurred, became particularly evident during the 1931 Scottsboro case, in which two white girls falsely accused a group of young black men of raping them in a boxcar. In September 1933, Warner Brothers released director William Wellman's *Wild Boys of the Road*, its trailer promising "The Living Truth About 600,000 Wild Boys . . . Innocent Girls! Driven to Vagrancy, Crime, Fates Worse than Death!" Moviegoers, however, found a stark depiction of the lives of three young hoboes—two boys and a girl dressed as a boy—who hit the rails in order to be "one less mouth to feed" for their hard-pressed families. They fall in with other young vagrants, endure rape and the loss of a leg, battle railroad bulls and police, and find shelter in hobo jungles like "Sewer Pipe City," where they eat around a communal stove. Arrested for attempted robbery, they're sent home by a kindhearted judge in a tacked-on Hollywood ending.

A more serious but no less graphic account of Depression wanderers came from a University of Minnesota sociologist named Thomas Minehan, who in 1932 donned some old clothes, went down to the freight yards, and jumped on a freight train. He fell in with a group of teenagers, both male and female, and chronicled his discoveries in a book called *Boy and Girl Tramps of America*. The culinary lives of Depression vagabonds revolved around missions, jails, and hobo jungles. Out in the sticks, jobless rail-riders found small-town America anything but welcoming. In one midwestern town, Minehan and his tramp friends were met by a cigar-smoking sheriff and nine deputies holding clubs made from ax handles. The tramps were promptly arrested and trucked to jail, where they received a meager supper of "one cup of cold tomatoes, mostly juice, one cold boiled potato with scabrous jacket still on, one slice of muggy bread."[5] As in most rural jails, local prisoners were treated far better than the "bums" from out of town. The following morning, resident criminals breakfasted on oatmeal with milk and sugar, two fried eggs with bacon, toast, prunes, a cookie, and coffee, while vagrants were served watery cornmeal mush and a dry slice of bread. Shortly afterward, the sheriff herded them back in the truck, drove them to a freight siding, and packed them in a boxcar heading to Chicago. This was known as "passing on," the traditional way that local governments across the country dealt with homeless migrants who arrived in their midst: ship them out of town and let them be the next community's problem.

Out in the countryside, however, tramps still found spots where farm families retained some sympathy for down-and-out vagabonds. Ten miles out of town, Minehan and a group of tramps jumped off the train at a spot known for a nearby quarry for swimming and a welcoming hobo jungle. Minehan and a pal found a farmer and his wife who let them dig up a couple of bushels of potatoes and gave them coffee and a generous farmhouse lunch: "Ham and egg sandwiches, buttered bread, two kinds of jelly, a dozen apples, fresh homemade cookies, and half a cake." After the vagrants helped with the chores, the farmer's wife also gave them three cabbages and all the apples they could carry. Their pals, meanwhile, managed to score fresh fish from a fisherman, three chickens, a chunk of salt pork, and milk. That evening, seventeen migrants, including two teenage girls, enjoyed a feast on a warm autumn evening:

> *Full of food and near a warm fire we are happy and content. There are lean-to's of willows and scrap tin to which we can retreat if it rains. No need to worry about cops and sheriffs, nor snoopy case workers at Welfare stations and hell-shouting ministers at missions. When it becomes colder we will have to follow once more the depressing routine of organized charity and be kicked from town to town, as we stand hungry and cold in bread lines, but no need to worry now.*[6]

As wanderers flooded the rails and roads, social workers attempted to both measure and respond to the transient crisis. In late 1932, a group of social work leaders estimated that the new vagabond army contained 200,000 boys and young men, as well as 25,000 families. A second census a few months later counted 1.25 million transients, including 145,000 girls and women, all living lives in peril. They also reported that the relief received by the roaming unemployed was at best woefully inadequate and limited by outdated rules about giving aid only to legal residents of a community. In April 1933, the *Nation* ran a four-part exposé on life in the "Starvation Army." At its end, the author predicted that "(1) Our country is in imminent peril of revolt; and (2) the revolt, if it comes, will originate with the wandering unemployed."[7] President Hoover had largely ignored this new wave of transients, with the exception of the Bonus Army. Now there was a new occupant of the Oval Office, whom social workers thought was both sympathetic and ready to take action.

Under President Roosevelt, New Deal administrators decided on a two-tier approach to dealing with the roaming jobless, one for youths and the other aimed at grown men. Roosevelt believed that a good cure for young wanderers was a little military discipline and some outdoor living. One of his first acts as president was to propose the creation of a "civilian conservation corps" that would give 250,000 young men the opportunity to live in rural camps and earn money planting forests and doing other outdoor work. Admission to the Civilian Conservation Corps, or CCC, as it became known, was at first limited to unmarried men between eighteen and twenty-five, including both young vagrants and unemployed men from regions near the camps. A few months later, veterans, including former members of the Bonus Army, were allowed to join. Various executive branch departments shared responsibility for the CCC, but the U.S. Army oversaw the camps themselves. The men, called "recruits," were first taken to army bases, where they were examined by doctors and then sent to the mess hall and told they could eat their fill: "The recruits, a large number of whom were thin-chested and emaciated, took the privilege literally and fully one-half took second helpings, marching up to the mess counter with their tin platters. The noon menu consisted of vegetable soup, roast beef with mashed potatoes, spaghetti with cheese, radishes and lettuce, strawberry pie, bread, butter and coffee."[8] Finally, dressed in their new CCC uniforms (actually World War I surplus gear), the men were shipped out to a CCC camp, usually in a state park, where they were put to work at healthy but demanding tasks in the great outdoors.

Life in CCC camps was run along quasi-military lines. After reveille at 5:45 a.m., the men trooped off to breakfast, which was cooked following the recipes of the U.S. Army's Quartermaster Corps. Rations were designed to be inexpensive and give enough fuel, at least 4,000 calories' worth, for a day of hard work. A breakfast could include bananas, cornmeal mush, hash, bread, butter, and coffee, while lunch, typically the heaviest meal of the day, might be Irish stew, coleslaw, cornbread, pickles, jam, and apple pie. One camp commander claimed the "forest soldiers" ate twice as much as regular army men, including a pound of meat a day and "huge tablespoonsful of potatoes and green vegetables, great hunks of bread and dessert." For their work, the men were paid $30 a month, of which they had to send $25 to their families (or, if they had no families, to a charity of their choice). The normal tour of duty in the CCC lasted six months, after which they had a chance to re-enroll, up to a maximum of two years. For many young men, the only problem with the CCC was gaining admission in the first place. In September 1935, the "forest army" reached a peak strength of 502,000 men in 2,500 camps. However, President Roosevelt, in one of his sudden shifts of New Deal policy, decided that balancing the budget took priority in the run-up to the 1936 election. Despite the fact that the CCC was the New Deal's most politically popular program, Roosevelt slashed its enrollment to 300,000 men and camps to about 1,400. Gradually weakened by bureaucratic infighting, poor morale, rebellion (particularly by African-Americans confined to segregated camps), and dwindling budgets, the CCC sputtered along until 1942, when it was finally disbanded.

For the problem of older migrants, the New Deal's solution was the Federal Transient Program, which started in mid-1933 under the auspices of the Federal Emergency Relief Administration. Like the CCC, the FTP was founded with high ideals and the best intentions. As with FERA's other relief programs, the FTP's rules were set by Washington but the actual work was done by state and local relief organizations. Before the New Deal, transients were the last group to receive relief under the old poor laws. Now the FTP funded a separate system of transient centers guided by federal regulations meant to guard against local governments' ingrained cultural biases against drifters and migrant job seekers. In rural areas, transients would be gathered into federal "concentration camps" (a term that had not yet gained its ominous connotations) designed for long-term stays. In cities, they would be directed to transient centers, where they could stay for a night or even a week or two. Over the next two years, the FTP opened more than five hundred rural camps and urban centers serving hundreds of thousands of transients. After the initial feeding and processing, travelers had the option of either continuing their journey, heading perhaps to rumors of a job or to stay with family, or remain in camp for weeks or even months. During that time, social workers worked with the transients to determine what skills, job advice, and so on they needed to again become productive members of society. Services in the camps varied widely depending on the competence of the administrator. One model camp was Camp Green Haven in upstate New York, with bunkhouses, a dining hall, a recreation hall, a laundry, a canteen, a tailor, an infirmary, a newspaper, a baseball field, a woodworking shop, classes in radio and car repair, and an eighteen-acre farm. Doctors, dentists, and optometrists made weekly visits to provide medical care, new teeth, and glasses for its residents. In return for room and board, men were required to work on construction projects, gardening, kitchen tasks, and the like.

According to Harry Hopkins, the FTP's official policy toward transients was that "the government will feed 'em and doctor 'em and sleep 'em. They can do the rest themselves. We won't bother them."[9] To attract wary hoboes and others suspicious of authority, the main draw of these relief stations was ample servings of wholesome food. Though amounts varied between camps, at their most generous the mess halls served as much as a hungry vagrant could eat. Indeed, one transient's meal resembled something out of Cockaigne, the mythical land of plenty, or in hobo terms, the Big Rock Candy Mountain, with its lake of stew and hens that lay soft-boiled eggs. In 1934, Edward Morriston, age twenty-five, arrived hungry at a New Jersey camp and went straight to the mess hall:

> For breakfast he consumed 32 hot cakes. At lunch, 14 breaded pork chops, several helpings of vegetables and six bowls of preserved peaches faded out of sight. And at dinner he disposed of 26 frankfurters, six bowls of sauerkraut and several portions of dessert. . . . He told the camp physician he hadn't eaten in two days and hadn't had a square meal in weeks. His normal weight, he said was 185 pounds, but he landed in camp weighing 120.[10]

In all transient camps, residents received three meals a day, generally costing between six and nine cents a meal and using many surplus foods. At Camp Del Rosa near San Bernardino, California, one day's menu included:

### Breakfast
*Stewed Fruit*

*Oat Meal and Cereal*

*Bacon*

*Scrambled Eggs*

*Fried Potatoes*

*Toast, Butter, Coffee*

### Dinner
*Lima Beans—Bacon*

*Cold Tomatoes*

*Pickled Onions*

*Bread and Butter*

*Tea*

SUPPER

*Hamburger Loaf, Spanish Sauce*
*Mashed Potatoes*
*Buttered Carrots*
*Pumpkin Pie*
*Bread and Butter*
*Coffee*[11]

The federal transient camps were a great boon to state and local governments that had neither the money nor the desire to take care of the Depression's army of wandering unemployed. Nevertheless, resentment began to grow against the program, spurred by newspaper articles with headlines such as "Leisurely Life at Ozark Transient Camps Agrees with Guests Who Stay On and On; Some Play Golf and Ping Pong."[12] Campers were portrayed as "weary willies" idling away their days and fattening up on the taxpayer's dollar. Although social workers lobbied strenuously for the camps, the program also lost the backing of the White House as the president turned against federal relief. Harry Hopkins also lost his cheerful paternalism toward the transients, saying, "There could be little doubt that what most of them needed was not casework, but a job."[13] In 1935, President Roosevelt shut down the Federal Transient Program along with the rest of FERA. Transients willing to work would be given jobs with the new Works Progress Administration, while the rest were returned to the care of state and local governments. However, wandering job hunters soon discovered that the WPA had few jobs available for them, while many communities, including New York City, refused relief to new arrivals because they were not legal residents. After the camps closed, transients again began begging in the streets, hitching rides out of town, and jumping freight trains to follow rumors of jobs, generous relief, and good weather. For many, their destination was the West, and principally California.

———

ON APRIL 14, 1935 a "black roller" of dust swept across Texas, Oklahoma, and Kansas. Blowing drifts of fine grit and poor visibility made roads and railways impassable and closed schools and businesses. People as far east as Memphis wore cotton masks to avoid inhaling the spreading plumes. One of the worst dust storms the region had ever seen, it certainly wasn't the first. This corner of the southern Plains had a semi-arid climate in which a few years of good rains might alternate with years of drought when dust storms were common. During the 1930s, however, human intervention combined with drought to create one of the century's greatest ecological disasters: the "Dust Bowl" that engulfed eastern Colorado, the Texas and Oklahoma Panhandles, and western Kansas. During the previous decade, a time of abundant rains, farmers had rushed to turn the region's grasslands into fields of wheat, using steel plows to cut and turn over the ancient prairie sod. They were much slower to adopt good conservation practices to preserve the thin layer of sandy topsoil from aridity and wind. A period of drought, the worst in memory, began in 1932 and lasted until the end of 1939. And every year, during the "blow months" of February, March, and April, the winds roared in and simply blew the land away.

Like most farm folk of that era, the wheat farmers of Oklahoma followed culinary customs that were closely linked to the land and the passage of the seasons. Even though most farmers earned a living off cash crops such as winter wheat (mostly red wheat for bread baking), they also kept pigs, milk cows, and chickens and planted vegetable gardens and fruit trees to fill the larder. In root cellars that doubled as tornado shelters, families kept mason jars filled with jams, pickles, and vegetables put up for winter, as well as potatoes and apples. As these supplies ran low in late winter, housewives looked longingly to the garden for the first shoots of onions to cure the family's "spring fever." When harvests were good, farmers enjoyed a diet rich in proteins, starches, fats, and sugar. The folk singer Woody Guthrie, who grew up in the farm town of Okemah, Oklahoma, remembered a typical meal of his early youth, a time of regular rains and large harvests, that included "beefsteak, thickened flour gravy, okra rolled in corn meal and fried in hot grease, hot biscuits with plenty of butter melted in between," and for dessert, sliced peaches from a can.[14] With a meal like that under your belt, it was hard to remember that every few decades the rains simply stopped coming, sometimes for years at a time.

When dust storms hit, the housewife's first task was to keep the dust out of the house and off the food. She sealed windows with tape and stuffed rags in cracks under the doors. She set the table with plates and cups upside down so they wouldn't catch the dust and kept the milk pitcher, syrup jar, and flour tins tightly covered. Still, the dust filtered through cracks and covered tables, clothing, skin, and hair with a coating of powdery grit. Family members began to cough and wheeze from "dust pneumonia" (something like black lung disease, but caused by silica-rich dirt), which could be fatal to children and old people. Out in the fields, dust and wind tore through the winter wheat, destroying the harvest and desiccating the soil so that vegetable seeds wouldn't take root in the garden. The combined effects of dust storms and the sagging farm economy ate into families' savings, forcing them to cut back on purchases at the town grocery store. They pared back their daily diet to the bare minimum of flour, lard, and potatoes, supplemented by anything they could glean from the fields. In spring, that meant shoots of Russian thistle, better known in its mature form as tumbleweed, which tasted something like spinach. For some reason, the population of rabbits spiked during the Dust Bowl years, so whole towns organized rabbit hunts, both to kill the pests that ate their meager gardens and to put meat on the table. After a few years of drought, poor harvests, and eating dust, many farmers fell behind on their mortgage payments, ran up big bills at the store in town, and finally decided to pack it in.

In May 1934, when dust from western fields began to fall on Washington, D.C., and New York City, the drought became national news. Reporters, magazine writers, and photographers descended on the southern Plains to produce dramatic, at times near-apocalyptic portrayals of abandoned farmhouses surrounded by encroaching dunes and cattle skeletons. In the spring of 1935, the journalist Margaret Bourke-White traveled through the Dust Bowl with a photographer and described roads filled with rattling trucks and Model Ts stuffed with people and possessions chugging West, the beginning of a new exodus:

> We passed them on the road, all their household goods piled on wagons, one lucky family on a truck. Lucky, because they had been able to keep their truck when the mortgage was foreclosed. All they owned in the world was packed on it; the children sat on a pile of bureaus topped with mattresses, and the sides of the truck were strapped with bed springs. The entire family looked like a Ku Klux Klan meeting, their faces done up in masks to protect them from the whirling sand.[15]

One of the most persistent myths of the Great Depression is that the Dust Bowl impelled a massive migration from the central farm states to the West. Between 1933 and 1940, roughly 400,000 migrants from the southern Plains and Midwest did enter California seeking jobs and land; many thousands more ended up in Oregon and Washington State. However, only 16,000 of those people crossing into California originated in the Dust Bowl region. The decade's black blizzards did impel many in the Panhandle region to pick up stakes, but they moved an average of only thirty miles, to settle in nearby towns or to double up with kin whose farms hadn't been so hard hit. Panhandle folk were stubborn and had seen hard times before; they would stick it out. The vast majority of rural migrants were dislocated by new technologies and changes in farm organization spurred by New Deal policies.

Beginning in 1933, the Agricultural Adjustment Administration paid farmers not to plant cotton, tobacco, wheat, and other cash crops in order to reduce harvest size and thus boost prices. If farmers were planting fewer acres, they naturally needed fewer workers to till the fields. Landowners were required to share their government money with the sharecroppers and tenant farmers who had worked their land, but in many cases they refused. They wanted to scrap the old-fashioned sharecropper system and convert their farms to modern agribusinesses tilled by tractors and financed with low-interest government loans. Big farmers literally starved out their tenants yet avoided punishment, with the collusion of sympathetic, largely southern AAA administrators. This was by far the most important cause of rural migration, from the northern Plains all the way to the Deep South. Exiled from their rickety homes, poor farm workers moved in two directions. Black sharecroppers from southern cotton plantations headed north to Chicago, Pittsburgh, Washington, D.C., and New York City. In the Midwest and southern Plains, white tenants and farm laborers piled their meager possessions into old trucks and headed down Route 66 toward California.

The great chronicle of that westward migration is John Steinbeck's 1939 novel, *The Grapes of Wrath.* Steinbeck was born and raised in Salinas, the main town in one of California's richest agricultural valleys. As a teenager, in the summer he worked alongside Mexican migrant laborers in the valley's sugar beet fields. As a mature writer, he chronicled life in California farm communities in novels such as *Of Mice and Men* and *In Dubious Battle,* the violent saga of a doomed fruit-pickers' strike. In 1936, the editor of the *San Francisco News* asked Steinbeck to write a series of articles on the new wave of migrants then starting to arrive by the thousands in California's inland valleys. The state's farm communities had long relied on Chinese, Japanese, Mexican, and Filipino workers to do their planting, weeding, and harvesting. The new arrivals, on the other hand, were what Steinbeck called "real" Americans, direct descendants of the men and women who settled the frontier. The following year, he retraced the migrants' journey along Route 66, and in 1938, in an astonishing burst of creativity, in less than five months he wrote his account of one family's trek from Oklahoma to California, which became the best-selling book of 1939.

*The Grapes of Wrath* follows the journey of the Joad family, cotton and corn sharecroppers from a farm near Sallisaw in far eastern Oklahoma. Like most sharecroppers from the southern Plains to the Deep South, their staple foods are salt pork, biscuits, cornbread, greens, lard, and coffee. During these hard times, however, with cotton at rock-bottom prices, they can barely afford to buy food. Their dilemma is memorialized in a sharecropper's song called "Eleven Cent Cotton and Forty Cent Meat":

> *Eleven cent cotton and forty cent meat*
> *How in the world can a poor man eat?*
> *Flour up high, cotton down low,*
> *How in the world can you raise the dough?*
> *Old slouch hat with a hole in the crown,*
> *Back nearly broken, fingers all worn*
> *Cotton going down to raise no more.*
> *Eleven cent cotton, eight bucks pants*
> *Who in the world can have a chance?*
> *Can't buy clothes, can't buy meat*
> *Too much cotton and not enough to eat.*[16]

As the novel starts, the Joads are being evicted. The landowner has bought a tractor and wants to maximize his acreage by plowing up every foot of his land, including the Joad home-stead. The Joads find a glimmer of hope in a handbill promising work in California. They sell their possessions, except what they will need for the trip, and buy a 1926 Hudson Super Six sedan, which they convert into an updated Conestoga wagon. Ma Joad, the family matriarch, then begins the task of organizing the family food supply. The men slaughter the family's two pigs, salt the meat, and store it in barrels. The chickens come along in a couple of coops. Ma Joad tells her son, Tom, what to take from the kitchen:

> All the stuff to eat with: plates an' the cups, the spoons an' knives an' forks. Put all them in that drawer, an' take the drawer. The big fry pan an' the big stew kettle, the coffee pot. When it gets cool, take the rack out the oven. That's good over a fire. . . . Take the bread pans, all of 'em. They fit down inside each other. . . . I'll fix up the rest, the big can a pepper an' the salt an' the nutmeg an' the grater.[17]

The men spend all night loading the truck, and at dawn the family breakfasts on coffee and roast pork bones. They all pile in; the truck roars to life and slowly lurches down the rutted road. When they reach the highway, they turn west toward the Pacific Ocean. They are optimistic about their future in California, but also wary—a conflict captured in a poem by an Oklahoma migrant named Flora Robertson:

> California, California,
> Here I come too.
> With a coffee pot and skillet,
> And I'm coming to you.
> Nothing's left in Oklahoma,
> For us to eat or do.

> *And if apples, nuts, and oranges,*
> *And Santy Claus is real,*
> *Come on to California,*
> *Eat and eat till your full.*[18]

Pushed by poor harvests, evictions, and generally hard times, the great wave of agricultural migrants such as the Joads began in 1934 and continued into the early 1940s. Most of those heading to California entered the state at the town of Needles, where they often were greeted by armed deputies. California had a long history of antagonism toward outsiders, going back to its early days as a territory. During the Depression, this hostility was exacerbated by the closing of federal transient camps at the end of 1935. Fearful of being inundated by hordes of "Okies," "Arkies," and "Texies," the Los Angeles police chief set up armed guards, also called the "bum blockade," at the state's main border crossings to turn back migrants. That ended a few months later, after it was found to be

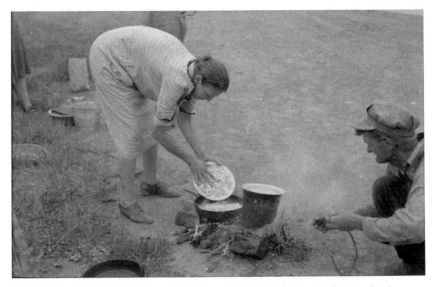

*Migrants on an Oklahoma roadside prepare a meal of potatoes fried in lard, 1939.* (Russell Lee photographer, Farm Security Administration Collection, Library of Congress, LC-DIG-fsa-8a26714)

unconstitutional. If California couldn't keep the migrants out, it would find myriad ways to make the state a less hospitable place to stay. The legislature tightened requirements for receiving relief from one to finally three years of legal residence. Many cities sharply cut back on aid to migrants. In Bakersfield, at the southern end of the rich San Joaquin Valley, the county welfare department would give transients only one meal, at best watery stew and stale bread, and ship them to the county line. The local Red Cross chapter had been told by the national office to give no food to transients, while the Salvation Army officer grudgingly fed any migrant who could find his house a mile out of town.[19]

The migrants who came to the San Joaquin Valley were amazed by the region's green grass in springtime, the flowering fruit trees, and ripe vegetables. However, as one migrant worker told a relief worker, "You can't eat the scenery. Even if it's 'most something to eat and you can't hardly enjoy the spring when you're hungry. But it is purty, ain't it?"[20] The dream had been to work hard and earn enough money to buy a few acres of valley land, build a homestead, and begin farming again. Instead, migrants discovered that no land was available; the valley had already been divided up into giant industrial farms, dubbed "factories in the field" by the writer Carey McWilliams, some covering thousands of acres. In the valley's economy, the migrants were useful only during harvest seasons; the rest of the year, they found themselves hounded from camp to camp by local police forces and goons on the big farmers' payroll. In *The Grapes of Wrath*, the Joads flee the squatters' camp after a fight with deputies, who torch the migrants' tents and shacks. Following a tip, they head south trying to find a "gov'ment camp" where, they've heard, they "treat ya like a man 'stead of a dog."

The novel's Weedpatch Camp is based on the government-run Arvin Sanitary Camp built southeast of Bakersfield. In 1934 and 1935, a group of federal relief workers, among them the economist Paul Taylor and the photographer Dorothea Lange, had traveled through rural California documenting the abysmal conditions suffered by migratory farm workers. They found a complete lack of sanitation, clean water, and decent shelter, as well as rampant infectious diseases and malnutrition. Moved by what they had seen, Taylor drafted a proposal, liberally illustrated with Lange's photos, for a string of migrant worker camps offering "healthful and conveniently located camp sites, adequate distribution of potable water and lighting throughout the camp, toilets, facilities for garbage disposal, bathing, laundering, and 'de-lousing.'"[21] Aware that relief money was tight, Taylor claimed that his camps would give migrants the "minimum decencies for healthful living"[22] while keeping costs low. With strong backing from his superiors, the plan eventually received a grant of $20,000 from the Federal Emergency Relief Administration and construction began on camps in Marysville in northern California and then in Arvin. John Steinbeck visited the Arvin camp while researching the migrants and relied on Tom Collins, the camp manager, as his principal guide into their world.

Although the migrant camp program was the brainchild of state relief workers, it was administered first by the federal Resettlement Administration and then by its successor, the Farm Security Administration. Even so, administrators back in Washington were stingy with both attention and funding. The camps were only a small part of the FSA's activities, which were focused mostly on giving loans and aid to farmers to keep them on their land in the first place. As waves of agricultural migrants spread across the United States, by 1940 the FSA had opened 56 camps around the country, 18 of them in California, each accommodating up to 350 families. Administrators nevertheless continued to keep costs as low as possible, following the "rehabilitation rather than relief" rule handed down by President Roosevelt. Rather than give migrants food, the camps taught home economics–style classes on nutrition and food budgeting. In a 1936 report from the

Arvin camp, manager Tom Collins reported how the classes had helped change the migrants' eating habits:

> *This week we noted a complete change in diet of most of the campers. The old reliable sow belly was missing excepting for breakfast. High prices had something to do with the absence of this staple from the daily menus. The discussions at the clinic and assembly of the "Good Neighbors" or women's club also were responsible. Fresh vegetables had a conspicuous place in the diets for the week. The change was beneficial, especially for the children. The use of vegetables has cut down the cost of menus.*[23]

This change was only temporary. During harvest season, when everyone had a few dollars in their wallets, the entire camp smelled like frying pork chops. And during the long months of no work, families lived on flour-and-water pancakes fried in lard.

As the numbers of migrants rose, relief workers like Tom Collins did their best to help the migrants despite a lack of resources and support from Washington. Community gardens were planted so campers could feed themselves—in the face of opposition from administrators who feared that having their own gardens would make campers less likely to move on. They opened cooperative stores in camps where migrants could buy healthful foods at reasonable prices. When strikes led to near starvation among California farm workers, managers convinced Washington to distribute surplus commodities such as flour, cornmeal, cheese, coffee, evaporated milk, vegetable shortening, and canned tomatoes. Still, the amounts given were a pittance compared to aid offered to resident relief clients: In February 1940, 3,511 out-of-state farm workers received $22,600 worth of surplus food, compared to $1.1 million of food given to 104,000 unemployed Californians.[24] That year, the FSA began a program of giving eligible families cash grants to pay for food and other necessities. However, the meager grants allowed migrants to buy only about two-thirds of the food necessary for an "adequate" diet. All of these efforts made a small difference, and certainly saved the lives of the most vulnerable, but they were clearly not enough to deal with a massive and growing problem.

Although California relief workers were able to help only a fraction of the thousands of needy migrants, they did have an outsize effect on the national debate about poverty and relief. In 1935, Dorothea Lange was hired by the Resettlement Administration (precursor of the FSA) to join its team of photographers documenting the lives of rural Americans. Early the following year, Lange encountered a group of destitute pea pickers camped in a muddy field near Nipomo, California. They had been stranded when a freeze ruined the pea harvest and were surviving on frozen vegetables from the fields. She talked to a tired young mother sitting in a ragged tent, little more than a lean-to, with her seven children, including a nursing baby. Lange quickly shot six photographs. A few days later, the *San Francisco News* publicized the migrants' troubles using Lange's photograph of the migrant mother below the caption "What Does the 'New Deal' Mean to This Mother and Her Children?" The strength of that image ignited a campaign to help feed the pea pickers, and within days they had received surplus food and help moving on to the next harvest.

Lange's photograph went on to have a life of its own. In 1936, the *New York Times* ran it twice as an illustration, once above a caption describing the subject as "a destitute mother, the type aided by WPA." It was widely reproduced in magazines and appeared in photography exhibitions, alongside the work of other noted FSA photographers such as Walker Evans, Arthur Rothstein, and Marion Post Wolcott. As it was reproduced and viewed by millions of Americans, the photograph "Migrant Mother" rose in stature. The hardships of an entire nation were projected onto that one image, which became the embodiment of motherhood, perseverance, and the American spirit. In the process, the photo lost its connection to its origin in a muddy field near Nipomo. Decades later, a writer tracked down the subject of the photo and learned her story. It turned out she was an Oklahoma native named Florence Owens Thompson, who had arrived in California during the late 1920s, married twice, and produced, eventually, ten children. To survive during the Great Depression, she and her husband followed the harvests; other times she worked in bars or restaurants or cooked and cleaned. By the time that surplus food arrived in Nipomo, the Thompsons had already fixed their car and moved on to another harvest. Florence never was helped by the WPA or any other relief agency, toiling in obscurity while her image became an archetype of Americana.

The other great depiction of Depression-era migrants, John Steinbeck's *The Grapes of Wrath,* was based not only on Steinbeck's reportage but also on the work of Lange and other FSA photographers, the images of *Life* magazine photographer Horace Bristol, Paul Taylor's studies of migrant life, and Tom Collins's information on the Okies' patterns of speech, customs, and beliefs. The novel, which was published in April 1939 to rave reviews, spawned dozens of newspaper and magazine articles on the Okies' hardships and, the following year, the Oscar-winning movie directed by John Ford. Eleanor Roosevelt, who had toured California migrant camps, gave the novel her wholehearted endorsement. But *The Grapes of Wrath* also had its detractors: it sparked an angry reaction among California farm owners, business leaders, and politicians, who painted it as a concatenation of lies, pornography, and Communist propaganda. They had a point—not all migrants received harsh treatment in California—but the novel hewed close enough to the facts, and the Joads were such powerful characters that it became (and remains) the dominant depiction of Okie life during the 1930s.

The furor over migrant workers led to a highly publicized investigation of interstate migration by Congressman John Tolan.

Hearings included testimony from the migrant farm workers themselves, big growers, social workers, labor leaders, and even Eleanor Roosevelt. After testimony spanning six months and hundreds of witnesses, the committee issued a damning 4,245-page report documenting terrible conditions faced by migrant workers across the nation and disorganized and woefully inadequate relief. At the very end, Congressman Tolan summarized his committee's conclusions. Rather than finding fault with migrants or with big growers, he pointed his finger back to Washington: "It all comes down to the question again as to whether the Federal Government owes a duty to people who are hungry or naked, or on account of circumstances over which they have no control are in need. Do we owe that duty or not?"[25]

# Chapter 10

—◦•◦—

THE WORKS PROGRESS Administration, led by Harry Hopkins, was among the most prodigious and lasting achievements of Roosevelt's New Deal. Its rationale was to replace relief handouts with jobs, allowing the unemployed to regain morale and self-respect. WPA workers were paid as employees, not as relief clients. Even today, the products of their labor continue to surround us. During the WPA's seven-year life span, its workers built, repaired, or improved 650,000 miles of roads, 124,000 bridges, 39,000 schools, 85,000 public buildings, 950 airports, 8,000 parks, and 40,000 miles of sewer and water lines. WPA-funded artists and writers performed 225,000 concerts and produced 475,000 works of art, from engravings to massive murals for public buildings and full-length plays, as well as 276 books. As direct relief ended, the WPA was ramping up operations, employing more than three million Americans by February 1936. Depending on the job, workers were paid a "security wage" of between $21 and $90 a month—less than they would have received for similar work in private industry but generally more than their old FERA relief benefits. By the time the WPA ended in mid-1943, about 8.5 million Americans had received paychecks from the agency, generally about 2 million a month until the end of 1940. WPA projects were distributed to every state, but the greatest were found in those with large relief populations such as New

York, Pennsylvania, Illinois, Ohio, and California. WPA jobs undoubtedly benefited workers, were a boon to numerous businesses that supplied raw materials for construction and other projects, and improved communities in every corner of the United States.

Unfortunately, the WPA did not alleviate the relief situation as much as Roosevelt and Hopkins had hoped. Many WPA workers discovered that they could not live on government wages, particularly if they supported large families. Also, WPA jobs lasted only as long as their projects, so workers often found themselves idle and counting days until the next position opened. In Baltimore, William Sutton received two months' work with the WPA, accepting a check for $24.75 every two weeks. Two weeks after he was laid off, the family bank account was down to $2, while the larder held only "four potatoes, a package of cereal, two loaves of bread, one-quarter of a pound of coffee, one pound of sugar and a can of milk."[1] In Denver and Seattle, where local relief was relatively generous, some workers found it made more sense to quit their jobs and apply for aid that would go further to feed their family. After all, one social work leader commented, "You can't eat morale."[2]

Another difficulty for the unemployed was that they were many and WPA jobs were few. In 1936, the unemployment rate was 16.9 percent, with about nine million out of work. The WPA could give jobs to about three million. What happened to the other six million workers, as well as their spouses and children? The Roosevelt administration believed that it was time for state and city governments to take up the full burden of giving food, clothing, fuel, and rent money. As responsibility shifted, many parts of the nation reverted to the old, underfunded, poorly coordinated relief programs administered by a patchwork of local, county, and state agencies. Seventeen states started professional departments of public welfare, but most others largely abolished their departments and left giving aid up to local communities. Many towns went back to the old poor laws under which the needy had to swear pauper's oaths and see their names published in the local newspaper in order to receive minimal help. Nationwide, the money available to the unemployed was only a fraction of what it had been between 1933 and 1935. During December 1934, $200 million was spent on relief; on average, three-quarters of that came from the federal government and one-quarter from state and local governments in roughly equal portions. Twelve states, mainly in the North, contributed more than 30 percent of relief costs, but some southern states provided less than 5 percent of the relief budget, with Washington making up the rest. By March 1936, the federal share was heading to zero, while the total monthly state and local government contribution remained at $50 million (and would never go higher).

Repercussions of new budget cutbacks could be seen on the kitchen tables of the unemployed. In Washington, D.C., which was governed by Congress, local administrators were forced to cut relief allowances by 25 percent. Families that had been receiving $30 a month for food, clothing, fuel, and rent now had to survive on $22.50. On the old allowance, they may have—barely—been able to enjoy an "adequate" diet, but the new allowance forced them down to "emergency diet" levels. In the South, cuts were even more drastic, 50 percent or more. Stories began to pop up on the inside pages of the daily papers, such as these collected from New Orleans:

> *Eva Killian, twenty-nine, was declared by physicians to be starving to death when brought by an ambulance to a charity hospital here. She had been living on coffee and bread. A child who fainted at school was found to have been without food for twenty-six hours. A woman and four children were found hiding in an empty house. An aged woman and her fourteen-year-old daughter, found rummaging in the scrap heaps behind grocery stores, are but two of hundreds engaged in similar searches.*[3]

In New Jersey and Pennsylvania, the misery caused by relief cutbacks was compounded by chaos in the statehouses. In both states, divisions were sharp between Democratic and Republican legislators who were unable to agree on funding statewide relief. Groups of hungry, unemployed workers marched on the state capitals in Trenton and Harrisburg. In Pennsylvania, they helped convince the legislature to pass a bill authorizing new funding for relief. In New Jersey, they occupied the statehouse for nine days but were unable to sway the Republican-dominated legislature. Relief money dried up, and any unemployed worker unable to find a WPA job was told to move elsewhere if he wanted to feed his family on government funds. Those who did apply for food relief were subject to the whims and prejudices of the local overseer of the poor, who often relied on his own racial biases to govern food distribution:

> *Six Eyetalians will live like kings for two weeks if you send in twenty pounds of spaghetti, six cans of tomato paste and a dozen loaves of three-foot-long bread. But give them a food order like this [$13.50, state minimum for six persons for half a month], and they will still live like kings and put five bucks in the bank. Now you ought to give a colored boy more. He likes his pork chops and half a fried chicken. Needs them, too, to keep up his strength. Let him have a chicken now and then and maybe he'll go out and find himself a job. But a good meal of meat would kill an Eyetalian on account of he ain't used to it.*[4]

In Hoboken, the "hard-boiled" overseer Harry L. Barck arbitrarily slashed relief rolls from two thousand families to ninety in just a few weeks, calling them either "chiselers" or too lazy to work. "I'm in favor of giving the old American pioneer spirit a chance to assert itself" was his rationale.[5] Although Republicans lauded Barck as a hero for exposing the "relief racket," his tactics were harsh even for a tough waterfront town like Hoboken. Under FERA, the state relief administration had distributed eight hundred quarts of milk a day in town, but Barck quickly stopped that handout. Two months later, a three-year-old Hoboken boy died of lead poisoning because he ate paint chips when his parents couldn't give him enough food on their $10.80 a month allowance.

---

FROM THE DAY FDR announced that the federal government was quitting the relief business, social workers, union leaders, and politicians with large numbers of unemployed in their districts had predicted disaster. Walter West, the head of the American Association of Social Workers, cautioned that present relief plans would leave many people without food: "Adding up what states can do, what local governments can do, what the relief provisions of the Social Security Act may supply when appropriations are made, and the tiny fractional resources available from private funds, the total falls far short of meeting the known needs of the situation."[6] On the grounds that work relief was the best and most American remedy for the ills of the unemployed, Roosevelt and Hopkins blithely brushed aside criticisms from their once-staunch allies. If anybody was going hungry, it was the fault not of the federal government but of "miserly" local politicians. Anyway, they trusted that the days of relief were almost over. After all, unemployment had dropped from a high of 25 percent in 1933 to 14.3 percent in 1937, thanks mainly to all the federal funds pumped into the economy by New Deal programs. Looking forward to the 1936 election, FDR also wanted to fend off Republican charges that he was a free-spending wastrel who was drowning the country in debt. In fact, Roosevelt had never been as comfortable with budget deficits as his enemies believed. He wanted to balance the budget and gave Hopkins and the other heads of New Deal agencies orders to immediately begin scaling back their programs. Hopkins slashed the number of people given WPA jobs from three million in early 1936 to less than half of that by mid-1937, despite thousands on the waiting list for relief work.

It quickly became clear that Roosevelt and his advisers had jumped the gun. In the late spring of 1937, the United States entered another sharp downturn, which Republicans labeled the "Roosevelt Recession." The stock market again plunged; factories closed doors; and hungry, unemployed workers crowded into relief offices. The years between 1933 and 1936 had merely been a lull in the storm; now Americans again felt the full brunt of economic collapse. In less than a year, the number of unemployed Americans jumped from 7.7 million to 10.4 million. However, Harry Hopkins only increased the number of WPA jobs from 1.45 million in September 1937 to 3.3 million in November 1938. Seven million unemployed workers, most of them supporting families, were stuck without any form of work, and beyond them were many millions of "unemployables" with few resources for supporting themselves. Somehow the lessons of recent history had not been learned, as the period between late 1937 and early 1940 was a return to the bad old days of the early 1930s.

IN 1938, THE American Association of Social Workers surveyed the relief situation in twenty-eight states and found that its prediction of hard times had come true. The number of WPA jobs was too small to go around, and where jobs existed, wages were too low to support families. Transients and aliens could expect little or no relief in most parts of the country. Many areas had nearly run out of relief funds, even after tightening eligibility, and periodically stopped aid altogether. Families faced widespread evictions because relief agencies no longer paid rent; thousands of children were barred from school for lack of sufficient clothing; and relief allowances were often painfully inadequate.

Reports of malnutrition across the country were rising. In April, a laborer named Samuel La Russo sat in the waiting area of a relief office on Bleecker Street in New York City, hoping to plead once again for help for his family. He had been on and off relief since 1934, but the previous year his name had been crossed off relief rolls for accepting aid while employed. Meanwhile, back in the family's tenement apartment on East Thirteenth Street, his wife and five children hadn't eaten in two days. The children had been crying all morning for food. Finally, their mother told them that she would feed them if they would first all go to bed and take a nap. She tucked them in, locked the front door, and then went into the kitchen and turned on all the gas jets on the stove. Within minutes, all of them were unconscious, except for the oldest boy, who staggered to the door and hammered weakly on it until a neighbor heard the noise and smelled the gas. She ran to get a policeman, who broke down the door and called an ambulance. The ambulance crew managed to revive them all, and doctors at Bellevue Hospital later said they believed they would survive, but their story was symptomatic of a larger desperation.[7]

White-collar families suffered from hunger as well. John Devlin, an unemployed accountant, and his wife were down to "three or four pieces of stale bread and two onions" to feed their two school-age children. They decided to apply for relief for the first time. After enduring the humiliation of the social worker's interview, they received an emergency relief check for $5.90: "I was incredulous. '$5.90? For four people?'" Three weeks later, after a home visit from an investigator, they received their first biweekly relief check of $14.20 to cover food, gas, and electricity:

> We had trouble learning to live within the food allowance allotted us. We learned it meant oleomargarine instead of butter. It meant one quart of milk a day for the children instead of three. It meant meat only twice a week—Wednesdays and Sundays.

*It meant a huge quantity of bulky, inexpensive vegetables. But,*
*somehow, we managed.*

*It was only after nearly three weeks had passed that I no-*
*ticed Joan was thinner. I didn't say anything at first, but stood*
*on the bathroom scales. In three weeks I'd lost a little over six*
*pounds.*

Concerned about his wife's health, Devlin took her to see the
family doctor. After questioning both of them, the doctor handed
over a prescription to give to the relief agency. Outside, the couple
unfolded the note and read: "Mr. and Mrs. Devlin are suffering
from malnutrition . . . and are in need of a diet high in carbohydrates, with an abundance of fruits."[8]

The relief crisis snowballed through the first months of 1938 as
factories, textile mills, and mines shut down. The federal government paid cotton and wheat farmers to mechanize their planting
and harvests; without work, sharecroppers fled to California or
the northern industrial cities. The situation was particularly dire
in Cleveland and Chicago, the largest cities in two states sharply
divided between rural and urban populations. In both Ohio and
Illinois, the state legislatures were controlled by Republican governors and farm-country legislators who had little sympathy with
the cities' largely Democratic, unionized, and immigrant population. In mid-May, local relief authorities in both cities ran out of
money to feed, clothe, and shelter their unemployed. In Chicago,
some 93,000 unemployed workers, most supporting families,
saw their direct relief vanish, while in Cleveland the number was
about 87,000. Hungry families crowded relief stations, clamoring
for food. A photograph that ran in dozens of newspapers across
the country showed men on a Cleveland street corner emptying
bags filled with potatoes into a big pile. One man used a shovel
to dump rations of potatoes into whatever container the unemployed managed to bring. Hundreds of grim-faced men, women,

and children in shabby coats and hats stood in line, holding boxes or pulling toy wagons that would carry their handout. One man said that he had sold his canary for five dollars to buy food, but now that money was gone. "I'm going to get something to eat," he said, "or know the reason why. I'm going down to City Hall with a gun." "Don't get yourself in any trouble," a woman in the crowd replied. "There's lot of grocery stores—go in and help yourself."[9]

Roosevelt and his aides kept a close watch on conditions in Chicago, Cleveland, and other cities. The president's initial policy was to do nothing and stay the course in the hope that the economy would turn around. His top advisers, meanwhile, agreed that something must be done but were sharply divided over what course to take. The Hopkins faction believed that a moderate increase in relief spending was in order, but all of that money should go to work relief, not direct relief. On the other side, those aides allied with Secretary of the Treasury Henry Morgenthau Jr. still

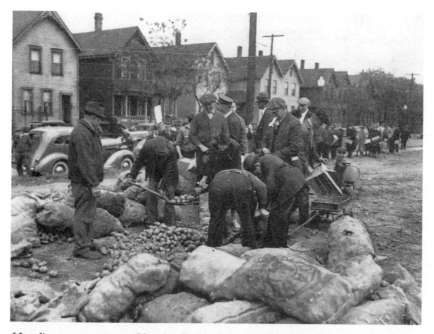

*Handing out potatoes to Cleveland's hungry unemployed, 1938.* (Authors' collection)

advocated the primacy of balancing the budget but wanted to take immediate steps to feed the hungry—using money already allocated for New Deal programs. As the bad news came in from Chicago and Cleveland, Morgenthau went to Harry Hopkins and asked him to release money from a WPA reserve fund to pay for food relief. Hopkins flatly refused. No situation, it appeared, was dire enough for him to consider returning to direct relief. Morgenthau next approached Henry Wallace, the secretary of agriculture, who oversaw the Federal Surplus Commodities Corporation (successor to the Federal Surplus Relief Corporation). Wallace believed his principal constituents weren't the unemployed but big farmers and farm state politicians. He saw the FSCC's main function as helping farmers alleviate crop surpluses, not feeding the hungry. Wallace refused to help, telling Morgenthau it would be bad politics. "All I could do was not to just curse in his face," Morgenthau told his aides. "I felt like saying 'I'm talking about feeding human beings, not hogs.'"[10] Despite Morgenthau's pleas, in June 1938 Roosevelt firmly closed the door on direct relief.

Instead, following Hopkins's recommendations, he asked Congress for emergency appropriations to aid those New Deal programs consistent with his favorite policies of work and farm relief. Thus the WPA, Civilian Conservation Corps, National Youth Administration, and Farm Security Administration were able to hire more unemployed. Larger numbers of WPA jobs helped some in Cleveland and Chicago, but the number of unemployed was always greater than available jobs. The FSCC also increased its distribution of relief food, but only if farmers, not the hungry, were the primary beneficiaries. What Morgenthau had hoped for was enough food to give the unemployed something approaching the old Holy Grail of an "adequate diet." They had received close to that in the early FERA days when relief boxes contained canned beef, salt pork, flour, butter, potatoes, tomatoes, cereal, cheese, and lard. Unfortunately, in 1938 beef, pork, flour, butter, and cheese were not being overproduced, and Wallace refused to purchase any food that was not in surplus. When the FSCC reluctantly released more food to feed Cleveland's hungry, handouts were limited to potatoes, cabbages, and butter. Chicago relief boxes contained dried beans, rice, cabbage, butter, prunes, celery, and oranges. Grapefruit was another common relief commodity, in fact so much grapefruit that people didn't know what to do with it. Serving suggestions for grapefruit began to appear in newspapers around the country, like this one from the *Atlanta Constitution*:

> *It may open the meal, served as a fruit cocktail, in halves with a spoonful of mint jelly in the center or sprinkled with a snow of powdered sugar. It bobs up in a fruit cup, or in a delicious ice. It may be served broiled with meat, appear in a fruit salad or in a grapefruit soufflé pie. Broiled grapefruit slices, seasoned with chili sauce, make an unusual and delightful accompaniment for broiled fish, baked fish or chops.*[11]

By the end of 1938, however, Wallace had decided to cut back on most surplus food handouts, preferring to pay farmers not to produce and to amass stockpiles of surplus commodities such as butter. The federal government's increased spending helped the economy recover—slowly—but the country still had more than ten million unemployed.

Although administered by Harry Hopkins, a critic of direct relief, the WPA did operate one program that fed millions of Americans: the national school lunch program. A holdover from FERA days, the WPA lunch program helped dozens of states pay for and organize hot meals in thousands of schools. The WPA had been under fire for giving few jobs to women; the school program allowed it to hire thousands of women whose only work experience had been as housewives. In the fall of 1937, however, Hopkins cut back hot lunch funds along with the rest of the WPA program, leaving the financing up to local communities. This was not always successful, as community leaders in Washington, D.C., discovered after they organized a gala "Velvet Ball" to raise money for school lunches that was so poorly organized that it lost rather than earned money. At the same time, the economy deteriorated, in many cases hitting children harder than their parents. Under pressure from Morgenthau and social work organizations, Harry Hopkins ordered the resumption of school lunch funding as part of an ambitious program to support students' health that also included doctors' visits, immunizations, and free eyeglasses. Between 1937 and 1939, the number of schools participating jumped from 3,839 to 14,075, covering almost 900,000 students.[12]

The federal financing of school lunches also became an avenue for dieticians and home economists to extend their influence far more widely than before. The home economics movement had always been interested in teaching children, particularly girls, the scientific basis of cookery and nutrition, but school dining rooms now offered them a new opportunity. In 1937, the American Home Economics Association adopted the following resolution:

> *WHEREAS, The school lunchroom is an important factor in child health and growth; and*
>
> *WHEREAS, Its administration requires a scientific knowledge of nutrition and professional training in institution administration; therefore,*
>
> *Resolved, That school administrators be urged to secure supervision of the school lunchroom by trained persons on a professional rather than a commercial basis.*[13]

If students would now be eating food prepared in school kitchens, they wanted home economists overseeing the staff and devising the recipes based on the latest knowledge in nutrition. They convinced hundreds of schools across the country to hire their own dieticians/home economists, while many others relied on nutrition and menu advice from home economists working for the local relief administration or nearby college. The WPA also assembled a small staff of home economists to make sure schools were serving "nutritious, well-balanced lunches" ideally consisting of tomato juice, a hot dish—soup, meat stew, vegetables, eggs, macaroni, or fish—a glass of milk, and a simple cooked dessert. The average cost per meal was a nickel. The largest school lunch program was found in New York City, where food was prepared in a massive central kitchen in Long Island City. Despite the need, teachers still had difficulties overcoming the ingrained tastes of students of disparate, often immigrant backgrounds:

> *Through years of patient persistence, children have been taught to like wholewheat bread, Spanish rice, cream soups, carrots and peas, peanut butter sandwiches and other dishes perhaps strange to them because not served in their own homes. While occasionally the educators have resorted to such tactics as coloring the once-disliked cream soups red with a little tomato, in the main they have trained workers just to be patient with getting children to taste dishes until they have gradually learned to like them. Children are also taught not to waste food. In some schools, proctors are appointed from older pupils to stand where trays are returned and report food that is not eaten. In the schools visited, plates came back as clean as a whistle.*[14]

Lessons in "eating American," it was thought, would not only breed good citizens but also improve the morale, scholarship, and health of the students. Beyond the dining room, home economists wanted to use the school setting as an opportunity to offer instruction in good behavior, sanitary habits such as hand washing, and "guidance in food selection in accordance with nutritive needs and economic resources of the pupils." Thus the cafeteria director would not only oversee lunch but also help the faculty to see the "health-teaching possibilities in all the experiences of the pupil's day."[15] The WPA's school lunches were meant to last only as long as the economic crisis, but home economists were determined to make them permanent.

By 1939, the problems of unemployment and what to do with millions of jobless Americans seemed intractable. The economy continued to sputter along; real prosperity remained an elusive goal; and Americans were losing compassion for the destitute and hungry. If people were still unemployed after nearly a decade of economic downturn, well, that was their fault, not the government's. In the 1938 elections, the Republican Party had made large gains in both the House and Senate and now wanted to both reduce the debt and cut taxes, forcing sharp cutbacks in all relief spending. Meanwhile, many mayors struggled to find the money to feed, clothe, and house their unemployed and a new wave of transients uprooted by the economic crisis. In many areas, the early New Deal benchmarks for adequate relief had been thrown out the window. A Houston, Texas, reporter lived for a week on the city's $1.20 weekly food handout, eating mostly oatmeal, potatoes, stewed tomatoes, and cabbage, and lost nearly ten pounds. In Chicago, a family of four received $36.50 a month, meant to cover food, clothing, fuel, rent, and everything else. But fuel in the cold Chicago winters was expensive; families had no choice but to cut back on food. In Ohio, the governor again refused to give aid to Cleveland, which ran out of money for nearly a month—called the "Hunger Weeks"—at the end of 1939. The city was reduced to feeding its poor with flour and apples as desperate families combed garbage bins for anything edible. Adults lost as much as fifteen pounds, while children had to stay home, too weak from hunger to attend school. Doctors saw a jump in cases of pneumonia, influenza, pleurisy, tuberculosis, heart disease, suicide attempts, and mental breakdowns.[16] A city nutritionist said that Cleveland would be "paying off years from now for sickness originating during the present relief crisis."[17]

For the hungry unemployed, the first modicum of relief began to arrive in May 1939. In yet another echo of the early 1930s, American farmers had again begun to produce far more wheat, cotton, butter, and other crops than the domestic market could consume. While prices plummeted, the farm lobby demanded immediate action from Henry Wallace's Department of Agriculture. Wallace ordered the AAA and the FSCC to purchase huge quantities of wheat and butter, but that only encouraged the farmers to produce more, exacerbating the new agricultural crisis. When Wallace proposed to sell the surplus to not only those on relief but also the working poor at drastically reduced prices, retailers protested because it would cut into their sales. Finally, Wallace fired his FSCC administrator and replaced him with one of his aides, Milo Perkins, with instructions to find a way out of the mess. Perkins worked with the big grocery associations to devise a plan that would both please retailers and farmers and help feed America's hungry.

On May 16, the FSCC's Food Stamp Plan was inaugurated in Rochester, New York, a "representative" city with about fourteen thousand on relief. Fifteen hundred unemployed citizens received their relief payments and then were given the opportunity to use that money to buy the nation's first food stamps, which were adorned with a portrait of "Miss Liberty" (called by some "Surplus Sal"). The orange stamps could be used at grocery stores to purchase anything but alcohol and cigarettes. For every dollar spent on these stamps, as a bonus the FSCC also gave recipients fifty cents' worth of blue stamps that could be spent only on surplus foods, also now distributed through retail groceries. During the first year, the surplus commodities generally included flour, eggs, butter, pork, lard, grapefruit, oranges, cornmeal, beans, hominy grits, onions, peas, canned tomatoes, and fresh fruits and vegetables. Over the next two years, the Food Stamp Plan was extended to cover more than four million Americans. People eligible for stamps included anyone on direct relief, all WPA workers, WPA applicants waiting for WPA assignments, and anyone receiving social security benefits, including the elderly and dependent children. Every week, they generally received a dollar's worth of orange stamps and fifty cents of blue stamps per family member. Six dollars a month for food was not much, but it was more than they were receiving from relief agencies in many cities. Administrators approvingly noted that most families used their blue stamps to purchase vitamin-rich eggs, butter, fruits, and vegetables. An Oklahoma physician described the program's effects on a rural Oklahoma family of eight:

> *Until the stamp plan this family was subsisting on whatever food the welfare agency had, sometimes nothing but beans. They got hold of some molasses, but no milk, no butter, meat or fresh vegetables; not even canned fruit. Here in truth was a* Grapes of Wrath *family. The children see-sawed between constipation and diarrhea. With stamps came health; the baby gained five pounds, one child three pounds, another seven.*[18]

The unemployed liked the stamps because they would not have to trudge to some far-off city commissary and could redeem them at any grocery store without the stigma of a handout.

The second boost for the unemployed came from a hiring spree by manufacturers, a development driven not by a change in domestic policies but by events overseas. In 1939, the menace of war that had hung over Europe suddenly burst into open conflict as Nazi Germany annexed Czechoslovakia and then invaded Poland in concert with the Soviet Union. The following spring, German forces resumed their onslaught, attacking first Denmark

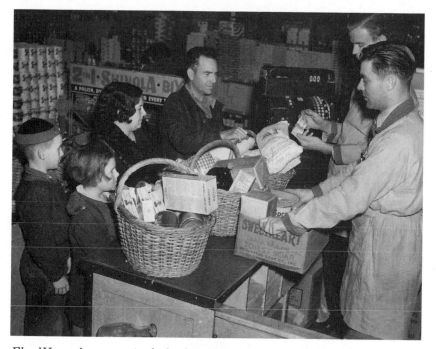

*Floyd Young buys groceries for his family, using the Los Angeles area's first food stamps, 1940.* (International News Photos, Corbis)

and Norway and then the Netherlands, Belgium, Luxembourg, and France. On June 14, when Nazi troops marched into Paris, President Roosevelt declared that it was now time for the United States to rebuild its military. Congress promptly increased the debt limit and approved the first of billions of dollars of defense spending. On the coasts and across the industrial heartland, dozens of enormous factories opened to produce guns, ammunition, tanks, airplanes, ships, chemicals, uniforms, and bombs. To man the assembly lines, these plants needed an army of workers— skilled, if possible, but if not they could be trained. The rumor of jobs unleashed a new wave of "defense migrants" converging on cities like Hartford, Detroit, and Seattle. Between San Diego and Los Angeles, seven vast new airplane factories put out a call for workers. Okies who had trekked to California dreaming of their own plot of land now turned their old cars south toward Orange County. Instead of tilling the soil, they found themselves in crisp new coveralls, punching a time clock. Between 1939 and 1941, the jobless rate dropped from 17.2 percent to 9.9 percent (and would shrink to 1.9 percent by 1943). The threat of war had done what neither President Hoover nor Roosevelt had been able to: solve one of the thorniest problems of the Great Depression.

The Roosevelt administration's rearmament program also called for a greatly expanded military to carry the guns, fly the bombers, and man the battleships. In September 1940, Congress passed the Selective Service Act, the nation's first peacetime draft. Two months later, the first conscripts lined up at induction centers, where doctors examined them to see if they were fit enough to become American fighting men. Government health experts remembered the debacle of 1917, when large numbers of draftees had failed their health examinations, but confidently predicted that 1940 would be different. Draftees would be taller and stronger, with good teeth and eyes and clear lungs; they expected perhaps 2 percent to be found unfit. They were shocked, however, when they tallied the figures: more than half a million draftees were examined, and 43 percent of them had failed. The culprits were poor teeth, bad vision, heart disease, syphilis, tuberculosis, and low body weight. Some military officers blamed the poor health on "soft living" and too much riding around in cars, but social workers placed the burden squarely on the Depression and the paucity of food:

> It is estimated that perhaps one-third of the rejections were due either directly or indirectly to nutritional deficiencies. The high rate of Selective Service rejections for physical disability points not only to widespread undernourishment, but also to other serious gaps in health protection. . . . While exact figures are lacking, it is clear that many of these young men could

*have passed their physical examinations if their defects had*
*been cared for while they were growing up. . . . Free school*
*lunches for children from underprivileged families, low-cost*
*milk schemes, and the "food stamp" system for distributing*
*so-called surplus foods have been tried out and have proved*
*of great practical value. But none of these methods is as yet*
*reaching all the needy people to whom this kind of food would*
*mean added health and strength.*[19]

In a second flashback to the Great War, reports had begun to arrive from Belgium, Poland, Finland, and other nations that starvation was again widespread across Europe. One country reputedly untouched by food shortages was Germany. If the German papers were to be believed, the Nazi army was efficient, tireless, and exceptionally well fed. American food experts worried that the Nazis had formulated some nutritional supplement, a "magical Buck Rogers pill," to energize their fighting men. Determined not to falter on the nutrition front, in May 1941, Roosevelt convened the National Nutrition Conference for Defense, which brought together nine hundred of the nation's top experts on medicine, nutrition, chemistry, education, and agriculture. At least a quarter of them were home economists. The president's letter to the delegates, read at the opening of the conference, communicated the urgency of the situation:

*Fighting men of our armed forces, workers in industry, the*
*families of these workers, every man and woman in America,*
*must have nourishing food. If people are undernourished, they*
*cannot be efficient in producing what we need in our unified*
*drive for dynamic strength. In recent years scientists have made*
*outstanding discoveries as to the amounts and kinds of foods*
*needed for maximum vigor. Yet every survey of nutrition, by*
*whatever means conducted, showed that here in the United*

*States undernourishment is widespread and serious. . . . We do
not lack and we will not lack the means of producing food in
abundance and variety. Our task is to translate this abundance
into reality for every American family.*[20]

Held at a Washington hotel, the three-day conference included
speeches by the surgeon general, Eleanor Roosevelt, and leading nutrition and home economics experts like Henry Sherman,
Elmer McCollum, Lucy Gillett, and Hazel Stiebeling. All acknowledged that the country was doing a poor job of feeding its
people. America's farmers produced more than enough food, but
too many people were too poor to buy it in sufficient quantities, or
lacked the knowledge to choose the healthiest kinds of foods. The
result was what one health expert was brash enough to define as
starvation: "Call it malnutrition, call it undernourishment, call it
dietary deficiency, or what you will—when men, women and children fail to eat the foods that give them full life and vigor, they
are in fact starving."[21]

Following the conference, delegates presented Roosevelt with
a long list of recommendations, including expansion of the school
lunch and food stamp programs. At the heart of their proposal,
however, was nutrition education: America would harness the
newer knowledge of nutrition to defend itself against the Nazi
threat. Scientists like Sherman and McCollum pledged to increase
spending on research, expanding the nation's knowledge of op-
timum human nutrition, while home economists planned a vast
new educational campaign. Ten years earlier, home economists
had seized on the economic crisis as their chance to make nutrition
relevant, but it now seemed their lessons had reached only a small
fraction of the country. The prospect of war had handed them a
second opportunity, and this time they would get it right. Clearly,
their teaching strategy would have to change. This time they would
be better organized and deliver their message in a zippier and more

appealing style. It was like the difference between classical and popular music, as one nutritionist said. Last time around, they had taken a classical approach; this time, it would be jazz.[22]

At a time when vitamins dominated nutritional thinking, it was apparent to everyone at the conference that they would be at the core of the new curriculum. A bit more fuzzy were the specifics of how much of which vitamins scientists would recommend. The goal was a "nutritional gold standard" in the form of a simple vitamin chart that anyone could understand. The night before the conference started, three women met in a Washington hotel room: the Bureau of Home Economics' Hazel Stiebeling; Lydia Roberts, the chairwoman of the University of Chicago Home Economics Department; and Helen Mitchell, a government nutrition scientist. Together, they pored over the most current research. By morning, they had compiled the first Recommended Dietary Allowances. Though hailed as a breakthrough—which in some respects they certainly were— their guidelines were strikingly similar to those formulated by Stiebeling years earlier in her *Diets at Four Levels of Nutritive Content and Cost*. The most salient difference was that Stiebeling now had the backing of the full medical and scientific establishment to lend authority to her nutritional charts.

As in earlier eras, the new guidelines were tailored to the individual's gender, age, and level of activity. They specified optimal iron, calcium, and calorie levels—up to 4,500 calories a day for very active men—but vitamins were the nutritional superheroes that would fend off disease and build strong bodies. Charts were printed in the daily newspapers with explanatory captions describing the special powers provided by each vitamin. Vitamin C not only prevented scurvy but also helped children grow, protected teeth and bones, and helped wounds heal. Vitamin D, the "sunshine vitamin," prevented rickets and regulated calcium and phosphorus levels to keep bones healthy. Vitamin A helped people build up resistance to infection and prevented night blindness (newspapers described how British pilots ate vitamin A–rich carrots to help them fight German bombers on nighttime raids). All were essential, but the vitamin with sex appeal was vitamin B, actually a complex of vitamins that then included $B_1$, $B_2$, and nicotinic acid. Now called $B_3$, nicotinic acid was the elusive substance which, when in short supply, was the cause of pellagra. Vitamin $B_2$, also known as riboflavin, promoted growth and healthy skin. The benefits of vitamin $B_1$—thiamine—were more elusive. Known as the "morale vitamin," $B_1$ was an overall mood enhancer. If you were tired, it added zip to your day. If you were a wallflower, it helped you get more fun out of life. If you were timid, it helped you live more intensely. If you were despondent, it gave you the will to live. All through the Depression, the Roosevelt administration and relief workers worried that government handouts would crush morale. Now with war looming, the nation's collective morale, enhanced by daily doses of vitamin $B_1$, would become a potent weapon in the American defense arsenal.

Home economists got to work promoting foods high in the B vitamins. Food columnists doted on liver and organ meats, not necessarily parts of the animal the public wanted to eat. Well, now it was time to get acquainted with them. Organs could be tricky to cook—prone to toughening up when cooked for too long—and were not pleasant to clean. Brains came in a transparent casing that needed to be removed, kidneys had an outer membrane, and hearts had to be divested of arteries and veins. In an organ meat roundup, syndicated food columnist Ida Jean Kain suggested scrambling brains with eggs; boiling kidneys with carrots, celery, and potatoes; and broiling heart with bacon. Chicago food writer Mary Meade liked kidneys on toast with a cheese and olive sauce. Liver was the most familiar of the organs. When combined with whole grain wheat, another of the B foods, the end product was a potent morale cocktail:

## Liver Loaf

2 pounds liver

4 slices bacon

¼ cup chopped parsley

1 onion

1 cup milk

2 flaked wheat cereal
   biscuits, crumbed

3 beaten eggs

salt and pepper

½ cup tomato ketchup

Method—Let liver slices stand in hot water 10 minutes; drain. Grind with onion, parsley and bacon. Add beaten eggs, crumbs and seasonings and pack firmly into loaf pan. Spread tomato ketchup over top of loaf. Bake one hour at 350 degrees. Garnish with broiled bacon slices.[23]

The germ of the wheat was where the vitamins resided. In the early 1940s, wheat germ popularity rose and even FDR went on record as a fan, adding a spoonful to his breakfast cereal. Wheat germ was also used in baking. "Marian Manners" of the *Los Angeles Times* helped lead the vitamin charge with recipes for liver loaf (above) and wheat germ spoonbread:

2½ cups boiling water

1½ teaspoons salt

1 cup cornmeal

1 cup wheat germ

3 tablespoons butter

1½ cups milk

2 egg yolks

2 egg whites

1½ teaspoons baking
powder

Method—Add cornmeal gradually to rapidly boiling, salted water. Stir in wheat germ. Add butter to hot cornmeal mixture and allow to cool. Add milk and slightly beaten egg yolks to cornmeal mixture. Beat egg whites until stiff. Add baking powder and fold into cornmeal. Pour into a greased baking dish or casserole and bake 40 minutes at 400 degrees. Yield: one 9x9 pan.[24]

With Americans in the throes of a newly discovered vitamin B deficiency, food manufacturers with products naturally high in B vitamins saw an opening and capitalized on it. Whole grain Quaker Oats made vitamin B the star of a snappy new advertising campaign: "I eat Quaker Oats for that wonderful extra energy 'spark-plug.' Jim thinks I have 'Oomph!' but I know it's just that I have plenty of vitality and the kind of disposition a man likes to live with."[25] What she did with her extra "oomph" was unspecified, but the graphic showed a young couple nose to nose, smiling into each other's eyes.

The vitamin B, or thiamine, shortfall was an unintended consequence of America's fondness for refined wheat and other grains, their vitamin content removed during milling and fed to livestock. For years, home economists had been praising the nutritional benefits of whole grains, but consumers were devoted to their squishy white bread and pure white rice. In recognition of consumer preferences, the big millers and bakers wanted to stick with their winning sales formula. When home economists suggested that their refined products were nutritionally lacking, manufacturers mobilized all their political might to protect the status quo. One way to please all factions, keeping profits high and consumers happy, was to add back in the vitamins they had removed. Sparkies, made by Quaker Oats, was one of America's first vitamin-fortified breakfast cereals, "spark" of course a reference to thiamine, the "sparkplug" vitamin. Launched in 1940, Sparkies were made from puffed wheat or rice, which, as the advertisements explained, had been showered with "Vitamin Rain." For advertising purposes, Sparkies teamed up with Little Orphan Annie and her new pal, a soldier named Captain Sparks, who could perform his daring rescues because he had eaten his vitamins. Home economists had wanted a jazzier way to sell nutrition, and now copywriters showed them how it was done in ads that used sex, humor, adventure, and also fear to get their message across.

Cereal was a good start, but America was then still a nation of bread eaters. Overwhelmingly the bread consumers ate was made from flour so milled and refined that it had been stripped of almost all vitamin content. In 1936, a chemist at Bell Laboratories discovered a method for cheaply producing thiamine, which quickly attracted interest from big bakers and millers. At twenty cents a loaf, about twice the cost of regular bread, the first enriched loaves were intended for the well-to-do when they hit the market in 1939. Early in 1941, the surgeon general announced that the government was developing standards for enriched white bread that would return a loaf's vitamin content to the level of whole wheat. As war approached, big mills and bakeries across the nation began to produce vitamin-enriched products. Ads for Ward's Tip-Top bread, which came in patriotic red and white wrapping, told homemakers to "serve that man of yours" the Tip-Top brand: "He's doing *his* job . . . working *in defense* of America . . . Do your job *right* . . . make *his* job *happier* . . . keep him *vigorous and fit* . . . with *well-balanced meals* . . . that's Health Defense at Home!"[26] The Silvercup bakery, an enriched bread pioneer, claimed that its new fortified loaf was "GOOD NEWS for the men on whom America depends," containing as many carbohydrates, proteins, calcium, iron, and vitamin $B_1$ as three pounds of baked beans, a nice steak, a bowl of cottage cheese, nine eggs, and a plate of calf's liver—and it only cost ten cents![27] If Silvercup was correct, people could forget about a balanced diet of milk, leafy greens, proteins, and carbohydrates, and face down all enemies on a regimen of enriched American white bread.

# Chapter 11

———◦•◦———

FOR ITS ROUGHLY two million readers, *Good Housekeeping* offered one escape from the worries of the Great Depression through the Shangri-La of modern domesticity that materialized every month in its pages. Since 1885, *Good Housekeeping* had been edifying middle-class women with uplifting poetry and prose. In the realm of nonfiction, articles on appropriately feminine subjects such as philanthropy, family, and education likewise cultivated what the publisher referred to as "the higher life of the household." For more practical enlightenment, readers could turn to the back of the magazine for lessons on such household arts as sewing, decorating, and meal preparation.

Over the decades, culinary instruction in *Good Housekeeping* evolved to reflect what was going on in the larger world, whether that meant a story on wheatless muffins during World War I or a 1920s tutorial on salads, the decade's "it" food. As the country entered the Depression, however, the clock at *Good Housekeeping* seemed to stop. Out of the hundreds of food stories published during the 1930s, only a small fraction were about economizing. In their place, articles with such titles as "The Importance of the Centerpiece" and "How to Prepare Delicious Hors d'Oeuvres" coached readers on the rigors of hostessing. Satisfying finicky husbands was another frequently visited topic. The magazine's advice: avoid second-guessing when feeding one's spouse. "It's bad news for a husband when his wife eagerly interjects, as the afternoon bridge players discuss new dishes: 'Oh, Harry wouldn't like that . . .'" Above all, however, the *Good Housekeeping* mission was apprising female consumers of the latest food products and kitchen appliances, all put through rigorous testing at the Good Housekeeping Institute.

The Good Housekeeping Research Station, forerunner to the institute, was founded in 1900 to help women sort through the growing marketplace of labor-saving devices for the home. Women confronted with such novel contraptions as gas ranges and washing machines needed protection against inferior goods and false advertising. *Good Housekeeping* proclaimed itself an impartial judge of the new technology. Before it granted its endorsement, every appliance featured in the magazine was put through its paces, tested not only for sound workmanship but also to verify that it lived up to the manufacturer's promises. More opportunity for consumer deception waited at the grocery market. As foods that had once been made in the home were increasingly handed over to factories, manufacturers turned to adulteration and misrepresentation to keep prices competitive. *Good Housekeeping* declared war on "dishonest food," rooting out products made with unsafe additives or cheap fillers. In a show of its integrity, only those products that had passed the testers' scrutiny were granted the privilege of becoming advertisers, and all products—national brands only, in keeping with institute policy—came with a money-back guarantee. A defender of the consuming public, *Good Housekeeping* was also a friend to the manufacturer. Anointing a product with the Good Housekeeping Seal of Approval imparted an aura of dependability invaluable to any brand, and products awarded the seal wore it conspicuously on their packaging. More fundamentally, though, the *Good Housekeeping* philosophy—that happiness depended on *things*—stirred a free-floating desire to consume that helped define American culture in the twentieth century.

Katherine Fisher, director of the institute during the Depression, was a home economist with a master's degree from Columbia's Teachers College, the same institution attended by Lucy Gillett and other prominent nutrition researchers. The institute kitchen, located in the New York City headquarters of the Hearst publishing empire, measured only ten by twelve feet, both floors and walls covered in the same blue and gray linoleum. Its size, however, belied its influence. In a decade of accelerated culinary change, the institute kitchen helped introduce women to a new strain of high-efficiency cooking built around the packaged and processed foods that advertised in the magazine. That included food that came in cans.

The first commercially canned foods appeared in the United States around 1820. Canned food really took off, however, during the Civil War, when hand-soldered cans of meat, peas, and condensed milk were supplied to Union soldiers. By the turn of the twentieth century, reports of illnesses—and even deaths—attributed to canned foods had been responsible for nationwide bouts of hysteria. Manufacturers were seen as unscrupulous, condemned for adding harmful preservatives and dyes to their products. The 1906 Pure Food and Drug Act was instrumental in cleaning up the industry and restoring confidence, but consumers still had to contend with a basic lack of product appeal. Canned vegetables were slack and tasteless, while canned meats and seafood were mealy textured and fruits discolored. Finally, canned foods suffered from the popular notion that only lazy housewives would resort to using them.

In the 1930s, *Good Housekeeping* worked hard to reverse that opinion. "Housekeepers are sometimes accused of serving meals 'out of the can' but today this is an outworn accusation," it reassured readers. On the contrary, the housekeeper who served canned foods did right by her family by feeding them "the best." Those with doubts needed only to review the modern canning process. Specially bred fruits and vegetables were harvested at the peak of ripeness—this was key—and processed at facilities right on the farms. Thus, foods served out of the can were "often fresher, and more healthful than so-called 'fresh' products" sold by the local green grocer.[1] Commercial canners were able to assemble the finest ingredients, maintain the highest sanitary standards, and employ master chefs. Really, how could a housewife compete? If canned vegetables still fell a wee bit short on flavor, which even *Good Housekeeping* had to admit was true, the institute had developed a special cooking technique to address that. For a "surprisingly full, natural flavor," it instructed housewives not to pour off the canning liquor but instead empty the can, liquor and all, into a broad skillet and cook over high heat until most of the liquor had boiled away, thereby concentrating flavor and nutrients.

*Good Housekeeping* also dismissed the old-fashioned notion that good cooking required hours at the stove. A Heinz advertisement that ran in the magazine both posed and answered the question:

> *Have you believed, as I used to believe, that the measure of a meal's enjoyment is determined by the pains and time involved in its creation? That every extra hour in the kitchen, added just so much more gusto to the feast?*
>
> *It is a theory somewhat less than cheering. For no matter how attractive one's kitchen may be, there are today simply scads of other things the modern household caterer must do.*[2]

Whether she worked outside the home or was simply busy inside it, the modern woman was by necessity an adept manager of time. In the interest of saving time in the kitchen, she happily availed herself of the convenience foods her mother had never known. The effect was like having one's own team of kitchen assistants. On rushed weeknights, canned foods were indispensable backstage helpers and the instant cure to that old bugaboo, monotony. The grocers' shelves held a multitude of possibilities:

*Canned fruit juices—grapefruit, pineapple, grape or tomato— ready in a jiffy for the first course! Delicious canned soups all ready to heat and serve in so many flavors that you can have a new one each night for several weeks! Canned salmon, tuna fish, sardines, crabmeat or shrimp—all so inspiring in hurried meal moments. As for old fashioned dishes like corned-beef hash, corned beef, codfish cakes, beef stew and spaghetti in tomato sauce, never let your family sigh for them, for we have approved several mighty good brands in cans, to say nothing of tongue, chicken and ham—all delicious enough to serve to the most honored guest.[3]*

When confronted with the same menu week after week, families were prone to sulk and might even stop eating, *Good Housekeeping* warned its readers. Variety pepped up "jaded appetites." Mixing two or more canned foods in a single dish multiplied a woman's quick-cooking options, an operation fully supported by the institute staff. Two different kinds of canned soup, for example, could be combined to make a third. Articles suggested mixing creamed celery and chicken soups, vegetable and bouillon, and tomato and consommé into "combinations every family will enjoy." By extending the mix-and-match principle, entire meals could be concocted from cans. Canned chicken was mixed with canned peas and shaped into a loaf. Canned spaghetti was sautéed with canned frankfurters, and canned shrimp were stirred into cream of mushroom soup—canned, of course—and poured over toast, thus eliminating the laborious and delicate process of making one's own white sauce.

Entertaining out of cans was permissible too. When guests

dropped in unannounced, a quick trip to the pantry "emergency shelf" held the answer to dinner. For ease of both preparation and cleanup, an all-in-one entrée was a godsend. *Good House-keeping* recommended a "Canned Kidney Beans and Frankfurter Salad Bowl," the two main ingredients combined with chopped gherkins and alternated with layers of lettuce leaves and sliced Spanish onion. Cold-weather guests might expect a warming dish of "Lima Beans De Luxe," canned beans bobbing in a pale yellow cheese sauce that was flecked with chopped canned pimento. For more festive gatherings, canned anchovies, olives, and sardines were served on crackers as canapés. For the salad course, canned fruits, all of uniform size and color, were arranged in eye-popping compositions. Canned apricots were stuffed with balls of cream cheese and chopped sweet pickles, served on lettuce leaves, and drizzled with French dressing. At holiday time, slices of canned pears, strips of green peppers, and maraschino cherries were used like mosaic tiles and arranged on the plate to resemble Christmas trees. More decorative still were the Technicolor "salads" that came to the table encased in flavored gelatin. The following is an example from the green family:

## Jellied Lime and Grapefruit Salad

1 package lime-flavored gelatin dessert
1 cup hot water
1 cup canned grapefruit syrup
1 cup drained grapefruit sections
½ cup sliced stuffed olives
Salad greens
1 avocado
Mayonnaise or French dressing

Dissolve the gelatin dessert in hot or boiling water, depending upon the manufacturer's directions. Add the grapefruit syrup, drained from the canned grapefruit; then cool until it begins to thicken. Add the drained grapefruit and sliced olives, turn into 8 small individual molds and chill until set. Unmold on salad greens arranged on a large platter, and garnish with slices of avocado. Serve with mayonnaise or French dressing. Serves 8.[4]

---

*Good Housekeeping* was a faithful advocate for the American food industry, but manufacturers had more direct ways of communicating with the public. Since the days of Fannie Farmer, food companies such as Rumford Chemical Works (which produced baking powder) and the Baker Chocolate Company had hired home economists to develop promotional recipe booklets using their products. During World War I, giant steps forward in the technology of mass production began to revolutionize both the food industry and the American diet. In the 1920s, as a new generation of scientific wonder foods appeared on grocery store shelves, manufacturers set up their own home economics departments to show women the merits of these newfangled foods. In the relationship between food producer and consumer, home economists functioned as go-betweens. They answered letters from customers, gave public lectures, and produced often-elaborate recipe booklets educating women in the many uses for products like Crisco and Velveeta.

A wave of corporate mergers in the 1920s produced the country's first food conglomerates. Businesses tied sundry food manufacturers into a national corporate structure; the new conglomerates combined sales, marketing, distribution, and research all under one roof, cutting costs and concentrating resources. In a field of giants, one conglomerate, General Foods, loomed over its competitors. How it grew to that stature is emblematic of the period. The company's origins go back to 1893, when a hardware salesman named Charles W. Post hatched a plan to invent a new breakfast drink. A former patient at the Kellogg Sanatorium and recent health food convert, Post was looking to formulate a caffeine-free alternative to coffee. The drink he came up with was Postum, made from a wholesome blend of roasted wheat and bran. Postum debuted in 1895, followed by Grape-Nuts in 1898, and a cornflake cereal called Post Toasties in 1904. Post's daughter, Marjorie Merriweather Post, was exposed to her father's business from an early age. As a girl, she licked labels for him and went door-to-door selling his products. At age ten, she was accompanying him to board meetings and tagging after him on factory tours. When he died in 1914, C.W. left the company to Marjorie, the daughter he had groomed in his image.

In 1920, in a special kind of merger, Marjorie Merriweather Post married her second of four husbands, E. F. Hutton. One outcome of this union was Hutton's departure from Wall Street to help expand the reach of his wife's company. The buying spree that would create General Foods began in 1925 with the acquisition of Jell-O, and within four years had engulfed more than a dozen other companies. Almost all of them were well-known brands, with the exception of a small frozen food company owned by Clarence Birdseye. A student of nature turned businessman, Birdseye had stumbled on the magic of "quick freezing" during a stay in Labrador. While ice fishing, Birdseye was intrigued to see that fish pulled from frigid water immediately froze stiff when exposed to extremely cold air. When cooked, moreover, they tasted as good as fresh. The explanation was the size of the ice crystals. Any food frozen at moderate temperatures forms large, sharp ice crystals that pierce cell walls and membranes, turning foods soggy when thawed. At the same time, enzymatic changes that take place during slow freezing give foods an off taste, vegetables being particularly susceptible. Freezing at subzero temperatures, on the other hand, creates small crystals that leave cells intact and preserves true flavor. Birdseye carried his discovery back to the United States and set up shop in the fishing town of Gloucester, Massachusetts, first freezing halibut and then expanding his line to include meats, poultry, vegetables, and fruit. Marjorie Post happened on a sample of Birdseye's handiwork—goose, according to corporate legend—during a stopover in Gloucester on one of the Huttons' many yachting expeditions. Struck by the commercial possibilities of a frozen foods line, she urged her board of directors to add Birdseye to the growing family of brands. After three years of deliberation, Postum finally acquired the patent to Birdeye's freezing process in June 1929. Following the deal, the Postum Company was renamed, and General Foods was born.

The logistical hurdles of bringing frozen foods to market took years to fully work out. Refrigerated railroad cars had been in use since the nineteenth century, but the extremely cold temperatures required by frozen foods—10 degrees Fahrenheit or below— meant that cooling systems had to be reengineered. Once the frozen cargo arrived at its retail destination, it required special low-temperature display cases, which in the early years few stores could afford. The last link in "the continuous chain of cold" was a related investment. Early home refrigerators were unwieldy contraptions. The cold compartment where food was stored was physically separate from the compressor, which was generally set up in an attic or basement. One of the first home models to reach the market, the 1918 Kelvinator made by General Motors, was comparable in price to a new car. Over the next two decades, dozens of brands entered the field. The refrigerator wars had commenced: Electric refrigerators competed with those powered by gas and kerosene, each model distinguished by the addition of attention-grabbing "extras." The Leonard Refrigerator, for example, came with a foot pedal latch so you could open it with your toe. The

Frigidaire had a moisture-controlled compartment to keep vegetables crisp. The Servel, capable of making one hundred ice cubes at a time, included a freezer compartment, a feature that soon became an industry standard. By the mid-1920s, elegant all-in-one models had replaced the old two-part machines. Refrigerators were admired as objects of modern beauty. In the words of *Ladies' Home Journal,* "the things are so completely nifty to look at, that to see one is to have a passionate desire for one." Consumer desire translated into booming sales that continued through the Depression, thanks to a combination of falling prices, installment buying plans, and aggressive advertising.

With the arrival of her first refrigerator, a woman who contemplated buying a waxed box of frozen lima beans now had the equipment to store it. What she still lacked, however, was the know-how to transform that icy brick into something you could serve to the family. Instruction came from the manufacturers. By the 1930s, consumer service departments that had started with a staff of two or three now employed up to fifty women. No longer just recipe writers, home economists helped corporations anticipate the needs and wants of their women customers. They vetted advertisements, recommended packaging, researched novel uses for old products, and contributed to the development of new ones. But while their job description had expanded, home economists kept up their dialogue with the American Woman. They continued to answer letters and to churn out instructional literature—booklets, pamphlets, charts, and magazine and newspaper articles—on how to cook with processed foods. By the start of the Depression, they had found a new medium—radio—spreading their message to an ever-widening audience.

The consumer service department at General Foods was established in 1924 when it was still the Postum Cereal Company. The first department head, Margaret Sawyer, was the former director of nutrition for the Red Cross and, before that, a dietician for the army. She took the job, thinking she could use it to help teach the public "the essentials of sound nutrition and the importance of wise food selection." A year after she arrived, however, the corporate focus shifted away from healthful eating. Not all of the company's newly acquired lines were especially nutritious, and, unlike breakfast cereals, many of them were "ingredient products" used in cooking. As the company evolved, Sawyer adjusted her lesson plan, talking less about health and more about food preparation:

> *We find that along with our food products must go a host of intriguing suggestions to increase their use, precise information about measurement of ingredients, about their proper combination and handling, and about temperatures, equipment and standards. This information should be set forth so clearly and so frequently that it controls the actions of the woman in the kitchen.*[5]

Products like Minute tapioca or Swans Down cake flour, both owned by General Foods, were judged not in their raw state but in the way housewives *used* them. It was important, therefore, that women use them correctly. Eager to discipline home cooks and regiment the cooking process, home economists demanded precision in the kitchen, a domestic science fixation going back to the previous century. But whereas founders of the movement had believed that discipline would ennoble kitchen work, corporate home economists discovered it was good for business. Training women to use accurate measurements, cooking times, and temperatures helped guarantee that products came out the way they were supposed to, increasing the likelihood that customers would buy them again.

Frozen foods presented a new teaching challenge. The Birds Eye line was unveiled in 1930 in Springfield, Massachusetts, where ten stores had been selected to carry the new brand. A home economist was on duty at each location to demonstrate the miracle of quick-frozen foods. By 1931, Birds Eye was in select towns and cities up and down the Eastern Seaboard. A troupe of home economists followed its progress from store to store, educating women in the ways of this revolutionary product. Whereas canned foods were close to indestructible, frozen foods demanded more delicate handling. *Important! Read complete directions at bottom of package before using!* was emblazoned on early Birds Eye cartons, the single most important source of product information. General Foods also published *The Birds Eye Cook Book* to answer basic handling questions: Must products be used on the day of purchase? *No. For future use, place unopened box in freezing unit of your refrigerator. Contents are good as long as they remain frozen solid.* Do vegetables require washing? *No. All vegetables are sorted, washed and trimmed, even spinach, which comes out of the box free of sand.* Must vegetables be thawed before cooking? *No. Just open the box and pop the frozen block into boiling water.* Must frozen fish be stored separately? *No. Frozen fish is odorless.*[6]

The 1930s were a singularly inauspicious time to introduce a packaged food that required expensive technology (a refrigerator) and cost more than either its fresh or canned counterparts. For most of the decade, frozen foods remained a luxury item. Unfazed by economic reality, the women's magazines were agog over them. The sanitary and attractive packaging; the uniform contents already cleaned, hulled, trimmed, trussed, and deboned, saving homemakers hours of kitchen preparation; the technology that captured freshness, abolished the seasons, and erased the limitations of geography, allowing a midwestern housewife to serve her family "fresh" fillet of sole—all of these qualities represented the cutting edge of culinary modernity. In anticipation of the Birds Eye launch, a 1929 story in *Ladies' Home Journal* envisioned futuristic markets equipped with great refrigerated display cases that ran the entire length of the store. Here, customers could choose among neatly stacked cartons of frozen fruits and vegetables, meats, and seafood, all of uniform quality. Shopping would be a snap. When the food columnist Mary Meade first sampled frozen food in 1934, she went into rapture: "I've just finished a week of adventuring with a dozen of the most delicious foods I believe it has ever been my good fortune to nibble on questioningly and then eat up joyously."[7] A weekend in the country gave home economist Marie Sellers a perfect demonstration of how effortless cooking can be when "science sets the table" and frozen foods take the place of fresh:

> On our arrival at the cottage the first things taken out of the box of groceries were some packages of quick-frozen meats and vegetables which were hustled into the refrigerator's largest freezing tray to keep frozen until needed. . . . As the days went by, out came the packages in the refrigerator's freezing tray; farm-fresh broilers as delicious as if they had just been bought from the farmer down the road, tender calves liver that seemed to have a special affinity for the bacon in its sanitary wrapping. Fresh peas, asparagus, and spinach followed one after another—each vegetable ready to be popped into boiling water, with no preparation nor even washing needed.[8]

Allied with the national media, the federal government, and food conglomerates, home economists were uniquely positioned to dictate where American food was heading. Their influence was felt in the city and countryside alike, as local food traditions gave way to canned-soup casseroles and Jell-O salads. But not without protest. Outraged by the direction American food had taken, in certain key cities a gastronomic counterculture had been galvanized into action.

HENRY LOUIS MENCKEN was a Baltimore newspaperman, an editor, author, and commentator on all things American. Among them was the state of the nation's cookery, which he called "the

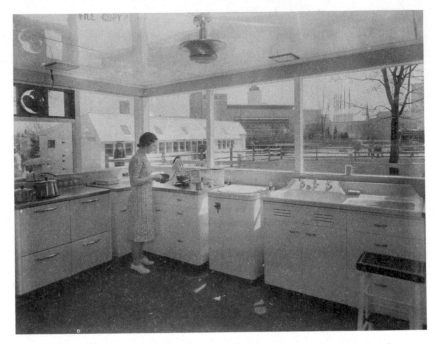

*During the 1939 World's Fair, a woman demonstrates the fully electrified farm kitchen. Well-lit, sanitary, and rationally organized, it heralded the modern food world to come.* (Manuscripts and Archives Division, the New York Public Library, Astor, Lenox and Tilden Foundations)

most subtle and kingly of all the fine arts." In the rush to become fashionable eaters, Mencken complained, Americans had cast aside native kitchen achievements such as Philadelphia pepper pot and southern fried catfish in favor of Continental slop. Across the nation, Pullman dining cars and hotel dining rooms served the same dull fare in whatever city you happened to find yourself. As regional specialties lost favor, gastronomes like Mencken were condemned to scour the streets of formerly great food cities for a decent plate of Boston baked beans or Baltimore steamed crabs. That was depressing enough, but then home economists came along, imposing their reign of culinary intimidation. According to Mencken, these domestic despots came in two types: Dieticians produced food that was nutritious but joyless, while "cooking school-marms" cared little about how food tasted but worried a great deal about how it looked. Both were enemies of what Mencken called "voluptuous eating." As a man who fought his battles with words, Mencken was rankled that home economists seemed to be the only people writing on food. To address the imbalance, as editor of the *American Mercury,* he put out a call for articles on the disappearing art of American victualary. A story on Pennsylvania Dutch cooking that ran in the *Mercury* exemplified what Mencken had been looking for: proof that in certain discrete pockets food traditions honed over the generations were still alive and well. Undeterred by dieticians, this rural community of German-Americans fearlessly indulged their gustatory yearnings with apple dumplings steamed over a pot of boiling ham, farm-made blood sausage, spaetzle seasoned with brown butter, hot sugary doughnuts, and syrupy shoe-fly pie dripping with molasses. Here was Mencken's voluptuous eating! Disappointingly, the article was just one of a handful on American cookery submitted to the *Mercury* during Mencken's tenure.

In the 1930s, the food counterculture found a new champion in a New York transplant named Sheila Hibben. Readers who came across her early food writing would have seen right away that Hibben was capable of bold pronouncements. Surely she raised some middle-class eyebrows when she wrote that anyone with an appreciation for honest food knows that "no virgin can cook really well." "To cook like an artist," Hibben explained, "there must be an experience of life—not of cook books—and a certain fecundity of feeling that cannot be dulled by routine and formula."[9] Here was the crux of the problem: American cooking was hostage to an all-female cabal of culinary technicians, women fixated on decorative salads, light entrées, and dainty desserts, nothing fecund about them. By the time she was forty, Hibben had accumulated abundant real-life experience. During World War I, she had served in France as a nurse with the Red Cross, for which she was awarded the Croix de Guerre. While there, she fell in love with her future husband, an American artillery captain and journalist named Paxton Hibben. After the war, the couple traveled to the Soviet Union on food relief missions, and finally settled in New York. In 1928, Paxton died of pneumonia, leaving Hibben to fend for herself and her six-year-old daughter. Several months later she published her first article, "Food Is to Eat," and in 1934 landed a staff job at the *New Yorker* as the magazine's first food critic.

But her reputation was made by *The National Cookbook* (1932), a compendium of regional recipes written at a time when the phrase "American regional cooking" was cause for puzzlement. *The National Cookbook* was conceived in a burst of culinary outrage, its source a picture in the *New York Herald Tribune Magazine* that showed a dog made of whipped cream—a terrier, no less—paddling across a soup tureen. The comestible canine, an example of the rococo assemblages favored by magazine editors, stirred in Hibben a renewed appreciation for the honest, savory foods that made up our culinary patrimony. For too long Americans had looked to Europe as the bastion of civilized eating. Hibben, who had spent years living in France, was well acquainted with the renowned foods of *la cuisine régionale* and felt the same honors should be paid to American regional fare. South Carolina hoppin' John, Pennsylvania pandowdy, and New England clam chowder were as good as anything found on the Continent. If native cooks had recently lost their way, *The National Cookbook* was meant "to call people home."

Hibben, like Depression-era nutritionists, saw economic disaster as an opportunity to mend our gastronomic ways. By the time the book came out in 1932, people accustomed to nights out on the town were trading in restaurant dinners for family meals and an evening gathered around the radio. As Americans amended their shopping lists and put their soup pots to work, some of the gastronomic freedom they had always taken for granted inevitably was lost. This was not all bad. "This depression, taking people back into the home, may have its silver lining," Hibben wrote. "Home-makers may begin to appreciate the simple, pleasurable dishes of their own country and serve them to their families. If that really happens, then this depression has not been in vain."[10] To cook simply and well, however, demanded certain adjustments in the ways people thought about food. Fifty years before Alice Waters, just as the variety of canned and frozen foods was soaring, Hibben was preaching the gospel of fresh and local ingredients. While magazine editors celebrated the defeat of seasonality, Hibben insisted we respect it. "We have been too spoiled," she wrote, "by a craze for food out of season; for peaches from South Africa and strawberries picked green and shipped too far."[11] The price for all that long-distance fruit was insipid pie and indifferent cobblers. Ingredients mattered.

At the same time, simple cooking required a more attentive cook. "The fundamental problem of the year 1932 is the question of economic adjustment—in cooks' terms, the problem of potatoes for all," Hibben wrote. "But, although this is fundamental, so also is a balance between what we have and what we make of it." In other words, it was essential that our potatoes should be boiled, baked, or mashed to perfection. With food anxieties rising, there was something fundamentally reassuring in Hibben's message. Food was to be enjoyed, and good food was within our reach. "Mink coats and period furniture are not always possible," she wrote, "but at least we can have omelets that are soft and melting, and soups that are savory and even beans that are succulent and satisfying."[12] While dieticians tended to our vitamin intake, Hibben was interested in the spirit-healing properties of humble food well prepared.

*The National Cookbook* made a splash not only in New York, where some of the city's most august dining establishments, including the Waldorf Astoria, began serving regional menus, but around the country as well. It's not often that a cookbook becomes fodder for reporters, but publication of *The National Cookbook* became a national news story. Under such catchy headlines as "Floating Dog Inspired Recipe Book," articles on Hibben and the glories of native cooking appeared in newspapers from Hartford, Connecticut, to Butte, Montana.

Still, Hibben must have been taken aback when she was summoned by Eleanor Roosevelt to advise the future first hostess on what to serve at the White House. In the months leading up to the 1933 inaugural, Eleanor had been reminded of an attempt by Martha Washington, another first lady who had lived in tumultuous times, to steer the country back to the simple, honest cooking befitting a republic. Eleanor wanted to follow her example. A woman whose relationship with food had always been more cerebral than visceral, Eleanor saw in Hibben a timely lesson about finding comfort in simple satisfactions. She welcomed, too, the opportunity to engage in some culinary boosterism, proudly showcasing historic American dishes made from American products to a beleaguered nation.

A month before the inauguration, Hibben sent Eleanor a sampling of historic and regional menus that she thought suitable for the presidential table. For a spring dinner she suggested a mid-Atlantic menu of calf's head soup, with a second course of planked shad roe and bacon, followed by fried chicken with cream gravy. Dessert was a strawberry blancmange. Her New England dinner started with Cape Cod clam chowder, moved on to corned beef and cabbage, and finished with a baked Indian pudding. There were breakfast and luncheon menus, too, fourteen in all. Hibben had hoped to debut one of them at the president's inaugural lunch, but was disappointed when Eleanor decided on tea sandwiches and jellied bouillon instead. After the inauguration, Hibben was invited to Washington to meet with Eleanor and the indomitable Roosevelt housekeeper, Mrs. Nesbitt. Over the

next several days, Hibben demonstrated for Nesbitt how to prepare hoppin' John, Martha Washington's crab soup, and gumbo
z'herbes, dishes that represented the American genius for honest
cooking. Some weeks later, Eleanor finally revealed to the public
that she was embarking on a Hibben-inspired culinary revival.
"The American menus of Mrs. Sheila Hibben," she told reporters,
"I hope will interest people not only in good early American food
but in the history that lies back of the recipes."[13] By this time,
however, she had already introduced the country to the Cornell
emergency diet prepared by home economists, which represented
a different strain of American cooking. Caught between the two
food initiatives, in the end Eleanor went with her progressive
instincts and chose science over tradition. Nonetheless, several
Hibben dishes, including calf's head soup and gumbo z'herbes,
a Louisiana specialty beloved by Andrew Jackson, were adopted
by the White House and served to guests. Years later, moreover,
when it was time for Mrs. Nesbitt to compile her own cookbook,
recipes for both of these Hibben dishes, along with several more,
were mixed in among the creamed casseroles and gelatin salads.
No attribution was given.

*The National Cookbook* foreshadowed another, even more ambitious ode to American foodways, this one produced by the
Federal Writers' Project. Created in 1935 under the auspices of
the Works Progress Administration, the Federal Writers' Project, along with similar initiatives in art, music, and drama, was
part of an experiment in the historically un-American activity of
government-sponsored cultural patronage. Intended to give jobs
to out-of-work novelists, reporters, and poets, in actuality the
writers' project employed roughly six thousand men and women
of highly variable skills and literary competence. Some were published authors and experienced editors, but "near writers," "occasional writers," and people who "probably can write but lack the
opportunity" were also eligible. Despite the ragtag character of

its hired hands, the writers' project managed to put out the enormously successful American Guide Series, a set of travelogues to each of the forty-eight states, Alaska, Puerto Rico, and the District of Columbia. Lewis Mumford called the guides "the finest contribution to American patriotism that has been made in our day," praise that was meant to silence critics who considered government forays into the arts yet more New Deal boondoggling.

The idea for the guide series came from Katherine Kellock, "a small tornado of a woman" who also served as one of its principal administrators. In 1939, as the series was winding down, Kellock began hunting for a follow-up project in a similarly patriotic vein. What she landed on was *America Eats!*, a region-by-region portrait of American cookery conceived in the same celebratory mood as *The National Cookbook*. In a departure from Hibben, however, Kellock's book would concern itself solely with the group feasts, church picnics, and grange suppers that were so characteristically American and that she believed were more resistant than everyday cooking to modern culinary influences. In her proposal, Kellock laid out, in her breathless shorthand, the book she envisioned:

> An account of group eating as an important American social institution; its part in development of American cookery as an authentic art and in the preservation of that art in the face of mass production of food-stuffs and partly cooked foods and introduction of numerous technological devices that lessen labor of preparation but lower quality of product.[14]

Hibben had told her story in recipes. By contrast, *America Eats!* would be not a cookbook but a series of culinary narratives, a multifaceted food ethnology punctuated by recipes and illustrated with photographs.

As to style, Kellock wanted the tone to be "light, but not tea shoppe, masculine rather than feminine," her way of asking for

writing with gusto—a word she resorted to often—both vivid with
sensory particulars and grounded in logistical specifics.[15] When describing group meals, writers should tell how they were organized
and who supplied the food. Examples of regional food disputes were
always welcome. Should the clam chowder contain cream or tomatoes? Should fried crabs be dusted with flour or dipped in batter?
These were the kinds of questions that food partisans could debate
for hours, a sign that regional food customs were matters of ongoing consequence. (Hibben, during her research for *The National
Cookbook*, was similarly encouraged by food partisanship.) What
Kellock hoped to avoid was typical frothy food writing. In fact, two
groups forbidden as contributors to *America Eats!* were professional
food writers and cooking school teachers.

It was up to Kellock to determine what foods were "American"
enough to deserve a place in the book. Sheila Hibben's defini-
tion of American food was expansive enough to encompass dishes
that were Dutch, German, French, Spanish, Scandinavian, Italian, Jewish, and Chinese. *America Eats!* took a narrower approach.
There were entries on Vermont Italian "feeds," Norwegian lutefisk
suppers, and the foods served at a Bohemian *sokol*. On the whole,
however, Kellock's understanding of what constituted American food was both highly selective and arbitrary. "Contributions
of national groups to the American table will be given attention,
though these are relatively few," she wrote in one of her memos.
After all, the purpose of the book was "to increase appreciation of
American traditions, and traditions brought to this country and
welded into the national life." *Welded.* That was setting a high bar.
The cuisines that qualified were German, Mexican, and northern
European. One Jewish meal, a Passover seder, found its way into
the manuscript, its presence justified "by the number of Jews in
the United States and the ancient character of the feast."[16] As an
example of the kind of immigrant group meal Kellock wanted to
avoid, she cited Chinese christening celebrations.

The "American" food traditions that Kellock instructed her writers to document were largely rural and coastal: threshing dinners, church suppers, cemetery cleaning picnics, barbecues, oyster roasts, fish fries, clambakes—and the list goes on. In the South, they encountered the food traditions of the region's African-American population, which was already the subject of a massive, ongoing writers' project. In 1936, field-workers for the FWP began interviewing elderly African-Americans who had been born into slavery and published their stories as *Slave Narratives: A Folk History of Slavery in the United States from Interviews with Former Slaves.* The *America Eats!* project extended that work into the realm of African-American food culture, particularly in the South.

Food was an occasion for gathering, whether coming together for a Savannah oyster roast or a creek-side fish fry. Conversely,

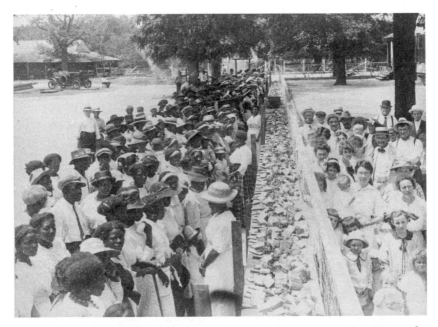

*Given yearly on an Alabama plantation, this barbecue was one of the communal meals that the* America Eats! *project set out to document. It also illustrated the profound segregation still prevalent across the South.* (Library of Congress, LC-USZ62-135594)

just about any gathering was yet another occasion to eat food together. So, a neighbor short on cash hosted a "Chitterling Strut":

> *These struts are held in the homes of the Negro for the purpose*
> *of making money to be used for anything from paying church to*
> *buying a winter coat. The meal is served on a long table reach-*
> *ing across the room. Wash tubs of cider sit on each end of the*
> *table where it is served with tin dippers. The pickle, slaw and*
> *potato custards are placed at intervals along the white cloth, but*
> *the chitterlings and corn pone are served hot from the kitchen.*
>
>     *The Negroes begin to gather by sundown. The host walks*
> *around barking*
>
> > *Good fried hot chitlins crisp and brown,*
> > *Ripe hard cider to wash dem down*
> > *Cold slaw, cold pickle, sweet tater pie,*
> > *And hot corn pone to slap your eye*
>
>     *By nine o'clock the feed is over and the shoo round strut*
> *begins. The table is pushed aside. The banjo pickers take their*
> *places back under the stair steps out of the way. With the first*
> *clear notes a high brown leaps to the center of the floor and cuts*
> *the buck. Couples form, then comes the steady shuffle of the feet*
> *and the strut is on.*[17]

---

FOR A HOST of reasons, *America Eats!* never made it into print.
For one, the quality of the material coming in from the field was
often disappointing. Memos from Kellock to regional editors are
full of phrases complaining that one writer or another "seems to
misunderstand the purpose of this book" or "can't understand that
this is not a cookbook." More issues arose from the high turn-
over in writers' project personnel and steady cutbacks in funding

arising from the Republicans' anathema to anything associated with the WPA and the arts. These kinks, however, might have been worked out, and the book might still have seen publication if world events had not intervened. The manuscript was due at the end December 1941, but on December 7 the Japanese bombed Pearl Harbor and on the following day the United States declared war against Japan, Germany, and Italy. As the FWP's staff was slashed, Kellock scrambled to cobble together a workable manuscript from whatever material she had at hand. But in May 1942, she was given orders to vacate her offices, while disparate pieces of *America Eats!* were boxed up and sent to the Library of Congress, to lie forgotten for half a century.

The food authorities who led America through the Depression were overwhelmingly white, Anglo-Saxon women. Not unreasonably, their ideas about food reflected where they came from, culturally speaking. Who but a WASP could think up a diet based around milky chowders and creamed casseroles? And wasn't Milkorno just a version of the same but with a scientific overlay? Another kind of authority, magazine editors, rejected their mothers' recipe boxes in favor of camera-ready cooking, food that was ready for its close-up but, as Hibben would say, missed the fundamental point that "food is to eat." Their sisters in the home economics departments of appliance manufacturers and food conglomerates peered into their crystal balls and liked what they saw: kitchens that were so efficient that food seemed to cook itself. Science, efficiency, technology, consumerism— this was the future. Point to any moment in American culinary history and you can rightly say, "Ahh, that was a transitional period." We are always coming from someplace to someplace else. During the Depression, however, the transition was especially stark. Afraid that our culinary heritage was in jeopardy, Hibben gave us *The National Cookbook.* The WPA's *America Eats!* project was another kind of gastronomic salvage mission, undertaken against the onslaught of modernity. Yearning for the past, an imagined golden age, before (you fill in the blank) came along and mucked things up, is a perennial occupation. Chances are that our own descendants will look back at the present era and wonder that we had things so good.

# Notes

## PROLOGUE

1. "Mauretania Arrives with 3,999 Troops from Overseas," *New-York Tribune,* December 2, 1918, 1.
2. "Welcome Home of Yankee Division," *Christian Science Monitor,* April 26, 1919, 8.
3. "While the Men Marched By," *New-York Tribune,* May 7, 1919, 13.
4. "Wants Holiday for Parade," *New York Times,* March 17, 1919, 5.
5. "4,000 Fed at 'Kitchen,'" *Baltimore Sun,* May 26, 1919, 2.
6. John Dos Passos, *U.S.A.* (1938; repr. New York: Library of America, 1996), 794.
7. Ibid., 805.

## CHAPTER 1

1. Country Life Commission, *Report of the Country Life Commission* (Washington, DC: Government Printing Office), 1909.
2. Gertrude Lynn, "The Step Saving Kitchen," *Home Economics Bulletin,* Iowa State College of Agriculture and Mechanical Arts, June 1924.
3. Elizabeth Ellam, "The Wife of the Farmer—The Woman God Forgot," *Boston Herald,* June 6, 1920, E1.
4. "Farm Women Who Count Themselves Blest by Fate," *Literary Digest,* November 13, 1920, 52.
5. Della Lutes, *The Country Kitchen* (Boston: Little, Brown and Company, 1936), 175.
6. Julie N. Zimmerman, *Opening Windows onto Hidden Lives: Women, Country Life, and Early Rural Sociological Research* (University Park: Pennsylvania State University Press, 2010), 177.

7. Ibid., 169.
8. Mary Meek Atkeson, *The Woman on the Farm* (New York: The Century Company, 1924), 302–3.
9. Edith Hawley, "Food Habits of Farm Families," *Nation's Health*, October 1926, 707.
10. Della Lutes, *Home Grown* (Boston: Little, Brown and Company, 1937), 168.
11. John Williams Streeter, "The Story of an American Farm," *Suburban Life*, April 1913, 251.
12. Eleanor Arnold, ed., *Feeding Our Families* (West Lafayette: Indiana Extension Homemakers Association, 1983), 92.
13. Adeline Goessling, *Making the Farm Kitchen Pay* (Springfield, MA: Phelps Pub. Co., 1914), 72.
14. "More Grape Recipes," *Angola Herald*, October 29, 1915, 2.
15. Arnold, *Feeding Our Families*, 92.

## CHAPTER 2

1. Townsend Ludington, *John Dos Passos: A Twentieth-Century Odyssey* (New York: Dutton, 1980), 197.
2. Ibid., 200.
3. John Dos Passos, *U.S.A.* (1938; repr. New York: Library of America, 1996), 789.
4. "Efficiency Apartments of Today Use the Fain Fold-Away Dining Room," *Building Age and the Builder's Journal*, April 1, 1924, 27.
5. "The Surf Apartment Hotel, Chicago," *Hotel Monthly*, December 1918, 50.
6. Isabel Cotton Smith, *The Blue Book of Cookery and Manual of House Management* (London: Funk & Wagnalls, 1926), 106.
7. Robert Kimball and Linda Berlin Emmet, eds., *The Complete Lyrics of Irving Berlin* (New York: A. Knopf, 2000), 196.
8. Jane Pride, "Kitchenette Workers of the Town, Unite!" *New York Herald Tribune*, July 6, 1924, SMA8.
9. Ibid., SMA8.
10. "Dining Out with Kitchenless New York," *New York Times*, January 25, 1925, SM4.
11. Raymond S. Tompkins, "Facts and Fancies Found in a Reporter's Notebook," *Baltimore Sun*, August 21, 1921, 14.
12. Brook Hanlon, "Delicatessen," *Saturday Evening Post*, October 24, 1925, 12.
13. "East Side, West Side, All Around the Town," *New York Tribune*, June 18, 1922, VI 3.
14. Ibid.
15. Florence Guy Seabury [née Woolston], *The Delicatessen Husband and Other Essays* (New York: Harcourt, Brace and Company, 1926), 28–29.

16. "Says Happiness Is Heart's Desire of Every Woman; High and Low," *Baltimore Sun*, May 1, 1921, 17.

17. George Jean Nathan, "The Sandwich," *American Mercury*, June 1926, 237.

18. *Soda Fountain Magazine* editorial staff, *The Dispenser's Formulary or Soda Water Guide* (New York: D. O. Haynes & Co, 1915), 27.

19. Display ad, *Detroit Free Press*, June 5, 1918, 6.

20. "Branzos Is Bran Plus Gluten and Fat," *New York Herald Tribune*, December 18, 1921, D13.

21. "Guide Posts to Balanced Meals," *Good Housekeeping*, January 1926, 64.

22. Thomas J. Allen, M.D., "Food Combination," *Medical Record*, July 2, 1921, 14.

23. Ibid., 15.

24. Antoinette Donnelly, "Diets That Bring Slimness," *Baltimore Sun*, January 31, 1926, MF1.

25. John K. Winkler, "The Man Behind the Pancake Front," *New McClure's*, December 28, 1928, 60.

26. Mrs. Christine Frederick, *Selling Mrs. Consumer* (New York: Business Bourse, 1929), 119.

27. Ibid., 127.

28. Ibid., 129.

29. Ibid., 129–30.

CHAPTER 3

1. "The Bread Line at Close Range," *New York Times*, February 16, 1908, C8.

2. Geraldine Sartain, "Bread Lines Here Longest Since '14," *New York World*, March 23, 1930, 15.

3. "Daughters of the Depression," *New York Herald Tribune*, August 9, 1931, SM4.

4. Meridel Le Sueur, "Women on the Breadlines," *New Masses*, January 1932, 5–7.

5. James K. Martindale, "Breadline Waste Hits at Families," *New York Evening Post*, January 10, 1931, 1.

6. Lillian Brandt, *An Impressionistic View of the Winter of 1930–31 in New York City* (New York: Welfare Council of New York City, February 1932), 5.

7. Ibid., 22.

8. Ibid., 8.

9. *Report of the Activities of the Mayor's Official Committee for the Relief of the Unemployed and Needy of the City of New York, October 31, 1930 to June 30, 1931* (New York: Mayor's Official Committee for the Relief of the Unemployed and Needy of the City of New York, 1931), 27.

10. Ibid., 28.

11. Frances D. McMullen, "School Relief Helps Many Families," *New York Times*, January 8, 1931, 117.

12. John Spargo, *The Bitter Cry of the Children* (New York: Macmillan Company, 1907), 107.

13. Martha Westfall and Josephine Adams, "Emergency Lunches in New York City," *Practical Home Economics*, March 1932, 99.

14. Martha Westfall and Josephine Adams, "The School Lunch as a Factor in a Health Program," *Practical Home Economics*, May 1932, 163.

15. Martha Westfall and Josephine Adams, "School Lunches as Part of an Educational Program," *Practical Home Economics*, January 1932, 22.

16. Ibid., 19.

17. Board of Education of the City of New York, *Thirty-Fifth Annual Report of the Superintendent of Schools for the Year Ending June 30, 1933* (New York: Board of Education, 1933), 229.

18. Allen Raymond, "City Teachers Add Relief to 3 R's by Raising $1,000,000 for Needy," *New York Times*, November 25, 1931, 1.

19. Brandt, *Impressionistic View*, 46.

20. Ibid., 40.

21. Ibid., 24–25.

## CHAPTER 4

1. "Farmers in a Good Position," *Ames Daily Tribune*, December 14, 1929, 1.

2. "Muscatine Men Expect Increase in 1930 Volume," *Mason City Globe-Gazette*, December 10, 1929, 9.

3. Lucy Rogers Watkins, ed., *A Generation Speaks: Voices of the Great Depression* (Chapel Hill: Chapel Hill Press, 2000), 253–54.

4. Lisa L. Ossian, *The Depression Dilemmas of Rural Iowa, 1929–1933* (Columbia: University of Missouri Press, 2011), xiii.

5. Wilma Walker, "Distress in a Southern Illinois County," *Social Service Review*, March 1, 1931, 568.

6. Ossian, *Depression Dilemmas of Rural Iowa*, 67.

7. "Broadcasting Home Economics from the U.S. Department of Agriculture," *Journal of Home Economics*, May 1927, 276.

8. "An Inexpensive Christmas Menu," *Housekeepers' Chat*, Washington, DC: U.S. Department of Agriculture, December 22, 1931, 1.

9. Ibid., 2.

10. Charles Morrow Wilson, "The Country Store Survives," *Outlook and Independent*, January 28, 1931, 142.

11. Tom E. Terrill and Jerrold Hirsch, eds., *Such as Us: Southern Voices of the Thirties* (Chapel Hill: University of North Carolina Press, 1978), 136.

12. "Oklahomans Barter in Wheat, One Tips a Waitress a Bushel," *New York Herald Tribune*, August 16, 1931, A11.

13. Rowena May Pope, *The Hungry Years* (Circle Pines, MN: Bold Blue Jay Publications, 1982), 35.

14. "Chicken Thief Came Near Being Caught at Johnson House," *Moravia Union*, August 28, 1930, 1.

15. "Loafer," *Denton Record-Chronicle*, December 4, 1930, 12.

16. Martin Gardner, ed., *Famous Poems from Bygone Days* (Mineola, NY: Dover Publications, 1995), 32.

17. "Recipients of Poor Relief to Be Published," *Kossuth County Advance*, February 4, 1932, 1.

18. Charles L. Dyke, "The Poor Fund Raid," *Sioux Center News*, August 25, 1932, 7.

19. "Tightening Up on County Aid," *Independent*, September 15, 1932, 8.

20. Marian Moser Jones, *The American Red Cross, from Clara Barton to the New Deal* (Baltimore: Johns Hopkins University Press, 2013), 43.

21. William D. Downs Jr., *Stories of Survival* (Fayetteville, AR: Phoenix International, 2011), 8.

22. Jones, *American Red Cross*, 227.

23. Nan Elizabeth Woodruff, *As Rare as Rain* (Urbana: University of Illinois Press, 1985), 27.

24. Ibid., 26.

25. Jones, *American Red Cross*, 233.

26. Woodruff, *As Rare as Rain*, 32.

27. Lement Harris, "An Arkansas Farmer Speaks," *New Republic*, May 27, 1931, 41.

28. Ibid.

29. "500 Farmers Storm Arkansas Town Demanding Food for Their Children," *New York Times*, January 4, 1931, 1.

30. Ibid., 21.

31. Ibid.

32. Woodruff, *As Rare as Rain*, 47.

33. Ibid., 48.

34. "Senate Defies Hoover and Votes $60,000,000 for Drought Relief," *Baltimore Sun*, December 10, 1930, 1.

35. Jones, *American Red Cross*, 229.

36. "Text of Hoover's Statement in Opposing U.S. Food Fund," *Baltimore Sun*, February 4, 1931, 2.

37. Downs, *Stories of Survival*, 50.

38. Ibid.

39. "Adequacy of Red Cross Feeding of Drought Sufferers," *Red Cross Courier*, February 16, 1931, 103.

40. William DeKleine, M.D., "Health of the People in the Drought Area," *Red Cross Courier*, February 16, 1931, 111–12.

41. Woodruff, *As Rare as Rain* 124.

42. Ibid., 111.
43. Ibid., 125.
44. "Hyde Gives Report on Drought Region," *Baltimore Sun*, April 8, 1931, 2.
45. Ernest Poole, *Nurses on Horseback* (New York: Macmillan Company, 1932), 8–9.
46. Mandel Sherman and Thomas R. Henry, *Hollow Folk* (New York: Thomas Y. Crowell Company, 1933), 42–47.
47. American National Red Cross, *Relief Work in the Drought of 1930–31*, (Washington, DC: American National Red Cross, 1931), 42.
48. Ibid., 153.
49. Theodore Dreiser et al., *Harlan Miners Speak* (New York: Harcourt, Brace and Company, 1932), v–vii.
50. "Calls Miner Serf in West Virginia," *New York Times*, April 3, 1931, 14.
51. "Says Red Cross Refused to Aid Starving W. Va. Coal Miners," *Baltimore Sun*, April 3, 1931, 1.
52. Woodruff, *As Rare as Rain*, 165.
53. "Payne Answers Barkley," *New York Times*, April 7, 1931, 13.
54. Mary Hoxie Jones, *Swords into Ploughshares* (Westport, CT: Greenwood Press, 1971), 225.
55. Woodruff, *As Rare as Rain*, 174.

CHAPTER 5

1. Walter I. Trattner, *From Poor Law to Welfare State: A History of Social Welfare in America*, 6th ed. (New York: Free Press, 1999), 22.
2. Emma Octavia Lundberg, "The New York State Temporary Emergency Relief Administration," *Social Service Review*, December 1932, 550.
3. "Underfed Children Problem in Schools," *New York Times*, December 23, 1917, 18.
4. Lucy H. Gillett, *A Survey of Evidence Regarding Food Allowances for Healthy Children* (New York: New York Association for Improving the Condition of the Poor, publication no. 115, 1917), 3.
5. Lucy H. Gillett, *Food Primer for the Home* (New York: Bureau of Food Supply, A.I.C.P., 1918), 18.
6. Helen Treyz Smith, "Budget Meals Can Be Good!" *New York Herald Tribune*, January 10, 1932, SM20.
7. Ibid.
8. Mary Meade, "Menu Planning Today Merits Extra Thought," *Chicago Daily Tribune*, February 13, 1935, E1.
9. Ibid.

10. "Dollar-A-Day Menus for Girls Planned by Y.W.C.A. Bureau," *New York Herald Tribune*, January 4, 1931, A14.

11. "Students May Live on 50 Cents Daily," *New York Times*, April 28, 1933, 19.

12. "Can Feed Four for $13 Week," *Ogden Star-Tribune*, November 23, 1930, 1.

13. Henry C. Sherman, *Child Health Bulletin*, November 1931, 185.

14. New York State College of Home Economics at Cornell University, "Menus and Recipes Prepared for the Temporary Emergency Relief Administration," undated, 4.

15. "Beggary Avoided in State Relief," *New York Times*, November 1, 1932, 3.

16. Eli Ginzberg, *The Unemployed* (New Brunswick, NJ: Transaction Publishers, 2004), 53.

17. Ibid., 51.

18. United States Senate, *Hearings Before a Subcommittee of the Committee on Manufacturers* (Washington, DC: Government Printing Office, 1933), 83.

19. William H. Matthews, "Cash Relief for the Needy Is Urged by Social Workers," *New York Times*, February 18, 1934, XX5.

20. Henry Hopkins, *Spending to Save* (New York: W. W. Norton & Co., 1936), 105.

21. Emma O. Lundberg, *Food Allowance Standards in the Up-State Welfare Districts* (New York: Temporary Emergency Relief Administration, 1933), 56.

22. Kathleen R. Babbitt, "Legitimizing Nutrition Education: The Impact of the Great Depression," in *Rethinking Home Economics: Women and the History of a Profession*, ed. Sarah Stage and Virginia B. Vicenti (Ithaca, NY: Cornell University Press, 1997), 157.

## CHAPTER 6

1. "Simple Fare Ends at the White House," *Daily Boston Globe*, January 23, 1929, B24.

2. Olive Ewing Clapper, *Washington Tapestry* (New York: McGraw-Hill Book Company, 1946), 4.

3. "Young Mother Is Victim of Hunger," *Piqua Daily Call*, December 16, 1931, 1.

4. "Starvation Victim Dies at Hospital, Too Weak to Rally," *Hartford Courant*, January 12, 1930, 4.

5. "Illness and Mortality Rates Cut Despite Depression and Idleness," *New York Herald Tribune*, August 22, 1931, 4.

6. "Nation's Health in 1931 Was Best on Record," *New York Times*, January 2, 1932, 12.

7. "Best Health Year on Record," *Sedalia Weekly Democrat,* January 8, 1932, 2.
8. Louis I. Dublin, "The Health of the Nation," *Better Times,* February 1, 1932, 5.
9. "Yes, There Is Starvation in New York City," *Better Times,* April 11, 1932, 5.
10. House of Representatives, "Unemployment in the United States," *Hearings Before a Subcommittee of the Committee on Labor* (Washington, DC: Government Printing Office, 1932), 98–99.
11. American National Red Cross, *The Distribution of Government Owned Wheat and Cotton* (Washington, DC: Red Cross, 1934), 32.
12. "Farm Board's Flour Arrives," *Los Angeles Times,* April 4, 1932, A2.
13. "Millions Fed by Federal Rations," *New Leader,* June 4, 1932, 13.
14. "Rebels of the Bread Line," *Irish Times,* May 10, 1932, 8.
15. W. W. Waters, *B.E.F.: The Whole Story of the Bonus Army* (New York: John Day Company, 1933), 6–7.
16. Ibid., 7.
17. Ibid., 14.
18. Gardner Jackson, "Unknown Soldiers," *Survey Graphic,* August 1, 1932, 342.
19. Waters, *B.E.F.,* 109.
20. Ibid.
21. Paul Dickson and Thomas B. Allen, *The Bonus Army: An American Epic* (New York: Walker & Company, 2004), 184–85.
22. Philip Brandt George, "A Dream Deferred," *American History,* June 2004, 38.
23. "Text of Governor Roosevelt's Speech in Boston Outlining His Program for Relief," *New York Herald Tribune,* November 1, 1932, 12.

CHAPTER 7

1. Louise V. Armstrong, *We Too Are the People* (Boston: Little, Brown and Company, 1938), 198.
2. *Manistee County Pomona Grange Cook Book* (Manistee, MI: Manistee County Pomona Grange, 1938), 23.
3. "I'm on Relief," *Harper's Magazine,* vol. 172, December 1, 1935, 202.
4. "Food and nutrition work of FERA reviewed with numerous state examples," FERA press release, July 15, 1935.
5. Catherine Hackett, "'Home Economics,' No Laughing Matter," *Forum and Century,* June 1933, 361.
6. John Steinbeck, *The Grapes of Wrath* (New York: Viking Press, 1939), 347.
7. Armstrong, *We Too Are the People,* 228.
8. Ibid., 264.
9. "How to Cook Salt Pork," Bureau of Home Economics, U.S. Department

of Agriculture in Cooperation with the Federal Emergency Relief Administration, Washington, DC, September 1933.

10. "Canned Meat Recipes," Bureau of Home Economics, U.S. Department of Agriculture, in Cooperation with the Federal Surplus Relief Corporation, Washington, D.C., August 1934, 1.

11. Lelia McGuire, "How to Buy Good Food Values on a Slim Budget," *Michigan Emergency Welfare Relief Administration News*, February 1935, 3.

12. "Milkorno Recipes," New York State College of Home Economics, February 1, 1933.

13. "Hopkins Points out Value and Extent of Subsistence Garden Program," FERA press release, New York Public Library, May 10, 1935.

14. Mary E. Dague, "Paradise Jelly," *Ironwood Daily Globe*, August 17, 1935, 3.

15. Letter from Edward J. Webster to Harry Hopkins, Harry Hopkins files, FDR Library, December 8, 1934, 5.

16. Josephine C. Brown, *Public Relief 1929–1939* (New York: Henry Holt and Company, 1940), 165.

CHAPTER 8

1. "Economy on President's Table," *Los Angeles Times*, March 2, 1933, 3.

2. Hazel K. Stiebeling and Miriam Birdseye, *Adequate Diets for Families with Limited Incomes*, U.S. Department of Agriculture, Miscellaneous Publications No. 113 (Washington, DC: Government Printing Office, April 1931), 2.

3. Rowena Schmidt Carpenter and Hazel K. Stiebeling, *Diets to Fit the Family Income*, U.S. Department of Agriculture, Farmer's Bulletin no. 1757 (Washington, DC: Government Printing Office, September 1936), 2.

4. "Vitamin Questions," *Housekeepers' Chat*, September 23, 1932.

5. "Using Whole Wheat," *Housekeepers' Chat*, February 17, 1932.

6. Bureau of Home Economics, U.S. Department of Agriculture, "The Market Basket," *Lincoln Evening Journal*, October 26, 1934.

7. "Dried Bean Facts," *Housekeepers' Chat*, January 15, 1934.

8. "Child Aids Listed by Mrs. Roosevelt," *New York Times*, May 2, 1933, 14.

9. "Mrs. Roosevelt Discusses Government's Aid to Home," *New York Herald Tribune*, November 18, 1934, A3.

10. Letter to Eleanor Roosevelt from Ruth Van Deman, December 4, 1933.

11. Alonzo Fields, *My 21 Years at the White House* (New York: Coward-McCann, 1961), 4.

12. Lillian Rogers Parks, *The Roosevelts: A Family in Turmoil* (Englewood Cliffs, NJ: Prentice-Hall, 1981), 69.

13. Laura Shapiro, "The First Kitchen," *New Yorker*, November 22, 2010, 78.

14. Michael S. Reynolds, *Hemingway: The 1930s* (New York: W. W. Norton & Co., 1997), 272.

15. Henrietta Nesbitt, *The Presidential Cookbook: Feeding the Roosevelts and Their Guests* (Garden City, NY: Doubleday, 1951), 103.
16. "Mrs. Roosevelt for President; No, She Replies," *New York Times*, March 2, 1937, 1.
17. James Roosevelt and Sidney Shalett, *Affectionately, F.D.R.: A Son's Story of a Lonely Man* (New York: Harcourt, Brace and Company, 1959), 237.
18. "Dear Neighbors," *Toronto Globe and Mail*, February 27, 1934, 7.

## CHAPTER 9

1. Eric Partridge, *A Dictionary of Slang and Unconventional English*, 8th ed. (New York: Macmillan Company, 1984), 557.
2. George Milburn, ed., *The Hobo's Hornbook* (New York: Ives Washburn, 1930), 218.
3. Nels Anderson, *The Hobo: The Sociology of the Homeless Man* (Chicago: University of Chicago Press, 1923), 35.
4. "Chicago Gets Shanty Town," *Los Angeles Times*, November 16, 1930, A7.
5. Thomas Minehan, *Boy and Girl Tramps of America* (New York: Farrar and Rinehart, 1934), 8.
6. Ibid., 16.
7. John Kazarian, "The Starvation Army," *Nation*, April 26, 1933, 473.
8. "Job Camp Army Puzzled, Happy at Camp Slocum," *New York Herald Tribune*, April 9, 1933, 16.
9. "Food, Shelter—and 90 Cents," *New York Herald Tribune*, August 5, 1934, SM8.
10. "Hungry Transient Offers New Peril of Treasury Raid," *Washington Post*, April 1, 1934, 2.
11. Ellery F. Reed, *Federal Transient Program: An Evaluative Survey, May to July* (New York: The Committee on Care of Transient and Homeless, 1934), 65.
12. "Leisurely Life at Ozark Transient Camps Agrees with Guests Who Stay On and On; Some Play Golf and Ping Pong," *Wall Street Journal*, May 2, 1935, 7.
13. Hopkins, *Spending to Save*, 133–34.
14. Woody Guthrie, *Bound for Glory*, 37th printing (New York: Plume, 1983), 42.
15. Margaret Bourke-White, "Dust Changes America," *Nation*, May 22, 1935, 597.
16. Ann M. Campbell, "Reports from Weedpatch, California: The Records of the Farm Security Administration," *Agricultural History*, July 1974, 402.
17. Steinbeck, *Grapes of Wrath*, 147.
18. James N. Gregory, *American Exodus: The Dust Bowl Migration and Okie Culture in California* (New York: Oxford University Press, 1989), 21.

19. State Relief Administration of California, *Transients in California* (San Francisco: no publisher, 1936), 60.

20. Sanora Babb, *On the Dirty Plate Trail: Remembering the Dust Bowl Refugee Camps* (Austin: University of Texas Press, 2007), 110.

21. Paul S. Taylor, "Establishment of Rural Rehabilitation Camps for Migrants in California," Emergency Relief Administration, State of California, 1935, 12.

22. Ibid., 12.

23. Thomas Collins, "Report for Week Ending April 25, 1936," Records of the Farmers Home Administration, National Archives, 5.

24. "Monthly Report, State Relief Administration of California," Sacramento: State Relief Commission, 1940, 46.

25. Kevin Starr, *Endangered Dreams: The Great Depression in California* (New York: Oxford University Press, 1996), 271.

CHAPTER 10

1. "Security Wage Misnomer, WPA Workers Indicate," *Baltimore Sun*, February 17, 1936, 4.

2. Gertrude Springer, "You Can't Eat Morale," *Survey*, March 1936, 76.

3. Isidor Feinstein, "Starving on Relief," *Nation*, February 12, 1936, 186–87.

4. "1936—Relief in New Jersey—1937," *Survey*, April 1937, 100.

5. Russell B. Porter, "Hoboken Slashes Its Relief Cases from 2,000 to 90 in a Few Weeks," *New York Times*, May 24, 1936, 10.

6. "The Relief State of the Nation," *Survey*, January 1936, 4.

7. "Hungry Mother Tries to Kill Self and 5 Children," *New York Herald Tribune*, April 15, 1938, 38.

8. John Devlin, "I'm On Relief," *Social Justice*, August 22, 1938, 13.

9. "Thousands Clamor for Food in Relief Famine in Cleveland," *New York Herald Tribune*, May 10, 1938, 1A.

10. Janet Poppendieck, *Breadlines Knee-Deep in Wheat* (Berkeley: University of California Press, 2014), 238.

11. Sally Saver, "Grapefruit Has Many Possibilities," *Atlanta Constitution*, December 4, 1940, 18.

12. Gordon W. Gunderson, *The National School Lunch Program: Background and Development* (New York: Nova Science Publishers, 2003), 22.

13. "The School Lunch," *Journal of Home Economics*, January 1938, 32.

14. "Lessons of Value in School Lunches," *New York Times*, January 9, 1938, N7.

15. Mary G. McCormick, "The Educational Possibilities of the School Lunch," *Journal of Home Economics*, April 1939, 228.

16. "Ravages of Crisis in Cleveland Told," *New York Times*, December 27, 1939, 14.

17. "Future Toll in Ohio Health Feared from Relief Crisis," *Baltimore Sun*, December 7, 1939, 1.
18. Don Wharton, "The Federal Food-Stamp Plan," *American Mercury*, April 1940, 478.
19. "Advancing on the Nutrition Front," *Social Service Review*, March 1, 1941, 560, 562.
20. "The National Nutrition Conference," *Public Health Reports*, June 13, 1941, 3.
21. *Proceedings of the National Nutrition Conference for Defense*, Federal Security Agency (Washington, DC: Government Printing Office), 21.
22. Helen S. Mitchell, "The National Nutrition Outlook," *Journal of Home Economics*, October 1941, 538.
23. "Marian Manners' Recipes," *Los Angeles Times*, July 11, 1941, A9.
24. "Marian Manners' Recipes," *Los Angeles Times*, May 2, 1941, A8.
25. "He thinks it's OOMPH! . . . I know it's energy," *Good Housekeeping*, March 1941, 162.
26. Display ad, *Chicago Tribune*, November 26, 1941, 16.
27. Display ad, *Chicago Tribune*, May 28, 1941, 20.

CHAPTER 11

1. Dorothy Marsh, "Canned Foods with New Appeal," *Good Housekeeping*, March 1930, 86.
2. Josephine Gibson, "Feasts Created Fast," *Good Housekeeping*, March 1934, 139.
3. Dorothy Marsh, "Dinners in No Time," *Good Housekeeping*, March 1936, 89.
4. Genevieve Callahan, "Entertaining Under California Skies," *Good Housekeeping*, July 1939, 151.
5. "From Food Factory to Consumer," *Christian Science Monitor*, May 24, 1932, 9.
6. Consumer Service Department, Frosted Foods Sales Corporation, *Birds Eye Cook Book* (New York: Frosted Foods Sales Corp., 1941), 6.
7. Mary Meade, "Quick Frozen Foods Are New and Practical," *Chicago Tribune*, January 12, 1934, 17.
8. Marie Sellers, "Science Doing Its Share in Aiding Cooks," *New York Herald Tribune*, September 27, 1936, K18.
9. Sheila Hibben, "Food Is to Eat," *Outlook and Independent*, March 20, 1929, 477.
10. Sheila Hibben, "Food Conscious Women Needed to Aid Depression," *Zanesville Signal*, December 25, 1932, 15.
11. Sheila Hibben, *The National Cookbook* (New York: Harper & Brothers, 1932), xi.

12. Ibid., xiv.

13. Villa Poe Wilson, "Mrs. Roosevelt Will Use Olden Presidential Menus," *Washington Post*, March 30, 1933, 1.

14. "America Eats," AE folder in Katherine Kellock file, Library of Congress.

15. "General Notes to Regional Editors of America Eats," WPA FWP, Admin File, A829.

16. "America Eats" file, Library of Congress, A829, Memo, October 16 1941.

17. Mark Kurlansky, *The Food of a Younger Land* (New York: Riverhead Books, 2009), 154–55.

# Bibliography

Abbott, Edith. "Unemployment Relief a Federal Responsibility." *Social Service Review*, September 1940.

Abelson, Elaine S. "'Women Who Have No Men to Work for Them': Gender and Homelessness in the Great Depression, 1930–1934." *Feminist Studies*, Spring 2003.

Adamic, Louis. *My American, 1928–1938*. New York: Harper & Brothers, 1938.

Allen, Frederick Lewis. *Only Yesterday: An Informal History of the 1920s*. New York: Harper & Row, 1931.

———. *Since Yesterday: The 1930s in America*. New York: Harper & Row, 1940.

American National Red Cross. *Relief Work in the Drought of 1930–31*. Washington, DC: American National Red Cross, 1931.

Anderson, Nels. *The Hobo: The Sociology of the Homeless Man*. Chicago: University of Chicago Press, 1923.

———. *The Milk and Honey Route* [Dean Stiff, pseud.]. New York: Vanguard Press, 1931.

Armstrong, Louise V. *We Too Are the People*. Boston: Little, Brown and Company, 1938.

Arnold, Eleanor, ed. *Feeding Our Families*. West Lafayette: Indiana Extension Homemakers Association, 1983.

Atkeson, Mary Meek. *The Woman on the Farm*. New York: The Century Company, 1924.

Atwater, Wilber O. *Principles of Nutrition and Nutritive Value of Food*. U.S. Department of Agriculture. *Farmers' Bulletin* no. 142, Washington, DC: Government Printing Office, 1910.

Babb, Sanora. *On the Dirty Plate Trail: Remembering the Dust Bowl Refugee Camps*. Austin: University of Texas Press, 2007.

Baker, Helen Cody. "What Is Starvation?" *Survey Midmonthly*, January 1940.

Bammi, Vivek. "Nutrition, the Historian, and Public Policy: A Case Study of U.S. Nutrition Policy in the 20th Century." *Journal of Social History*, Summer 1981.

Beals, Carleton. "Migs: America's Shantytown on Wheels." *Forum and Century*, January 1938.

Bellush, Bernard. *Franklin D. Roosevelt as Governor of New York*. New York: Columbia University Press, 1955.

Bernstein, Irving. *The Lean Years*. Boston: Houghton Mifflin Company, 1960.

Betters, Paul V. *The Bureau of Home Economics: Its History, Activities and Organization*. Washington, DC: The Brookings Institution, 1930.

*Better Times*. "Bread Lines Feed the Jobless." April 7, 1930.

Bird, Caroline. *The Invisible Scar*. New York: David McKay Company, Inc., 1966.

Bliven, Bruce. "No Money, No Work." *New Republic*, November 19, 1930.

Bonnifield, Paul. *The Dust Bowl: Men, Dirt, and Depression*. Albuquerque: University of New Mexico Press, 1979.

Bourke-White, Margaret. "Dust Changes America." *Nation*, May 22, 1935.

Brandt, Lillian. *An Impressionistic View of the Winter of 1930–31 in New York City*. New York: Welfare Council of New York City, February 1932.

Brown, Josephine C. *Public Relief, 1929–1939*. New York: Henry Holt and Company, 1940.

Bruère, Martha Bensley, and Robert W. Bruère. *Increasing Home Efficiency*. New York: Macmillan Company, 1912.

Bryan, Mary de Garmo. *The School Cafeteria*. New York: F. S. Crofts & Co., 1936.

Campbell, Ann M. "Reports from Weedpatch, California: The Records of the Farm Security Administration." *Agricultural History*, July 1974.

Cannon, Brian Q. "'Keep on a-goin': Life and Social Interaction in a New Deal Farm Labor Camp." *Agricultural History*, Winter 1996.

Carlson, Barbara. *History and Analysis of Food Guides in the United States*. PhD diss., Old Dominion University, 1991.

Carpenter, Rowena S. "National Nutrition Conference for Defense." *Scientific Monthly*, July 1941.

Charles, Searle F. *Minister of Relief, Harry Hopkins and the Depression*. Syracuse, NY: Syracuse University Press, 1963.

Chase, Stuart. "The Nemesis of American Business." *Harper's Magazine*, July 1930.

———. *Prosperity, Fact or Myth*. New York: Charles Boni, 1929.

———. *The Road We Are Traveling*. New York: The Twentieth Century Fund, 1942.

Child, Georgie Boynton. *The Efficient Kitchen*. New York: Robert M. McBride & Company, 1915.

Clements, Kendrick A. *The Life of Herbert Hoover: Imperfect Visionary, 1918–1928*. New York: Palgrave Macmillan, 2010.

Colcord, Joanna C., comp. *Community Planning in Unemployment Situations*. New York: Russell Sage Foundation, 1930.

Colcord, Joanna C. "Stamps to Move the Surplus." *Survey Midmonthly.* October 1939.

Coleman, McAlister. "Study in Relief." *Nation,* January 28, 1939.

*Compass.* "1938 Survey of Relief Situation." April 1938.

Cook, Blanche Wiesen. *Eleanor Roosevelt.* New York: Viking, 1992.

Country Life Commission. *Report of the Country Life Commission.* Washington, DC: Government Printing Office, 1909.

Cowan, Ruth Schwartz. *More Work for Mother: The Ironies of Household Technology from the Open Hearth to the Microwave.* New York: Basic Books, 1983.

Craig, Hazel T. *The History of Home Economics.* New York: Practical Home Economics, 1946.

Crawford, Ina Z. *The Use of Time by Farm Women.* University of Idaho, Agricultural Experiment Station, Bulletin no. 146, January 1927.

Cross, William T., and Dorothy E. Cross. *Newcomers and Nomads in California.* Stanford, CA: Stanford University Press, 1937.

Cummings, Richard Osborn. *The American and His Food.* Chicago: University of Chicago Press, 1940.

Dahlberg, Edward. "Hunger on the March." *Nation,* December 28, 1932.

Daniels, Roger. *The Bonus March: An Episode of the Great Depression.* Westport, CT: Greenwood Publishing Corporation, 1971.

Davis, Kenneth S. *FDR: The New York Years.* New York: Random House, 1985.

Davis, Maxine. "Hungry Children." *Atlantic Monthly,* January 1937.

———. *They Shall Not Want.* New York: Macmillan Company, 1937.

Dees, Jesse Walter, Jr. *Flophouse.* Francestown, NH: Marshall Jones Company, 1948.

DePastino, Todd. *Citizen Hobo: How a Century of Homelessness Shaped America.* Chicago: University of Chicago Press, 2003.

Devlin, John. "I'm On Relief." *Social Justice,* August 22, 1938.

Dickins, Dorothy. *A Nutrition Investigation of Negro Tenants in the Yazoo-Mississippi Delta.* Starkville: Mississippi Agricultural Experiment Station, August 1928.

Dickson, Paul, and Thomas B. Allen. *The Bonus Army: An American Epic.* New York: Walker & Company, 2004.

Dos Passos, John. *The Big Money.* New York: Library of America, 1996.

Dupont, Jacqueline L., and Alfred E. Harper. "Reflections: Hazel Katherine Stiebeling (1896–1989)." *Nutrition Reviews,* October 2002.

East, Anna Merritt. *Kitchenette Cookery.* Boston: Little, Brown and Company, 1917.

Elias, Megan J. *Stir It Up: Home Economics in American Culture.* Philadelphia: University of Pennsylvania Press, 2008.

Ellis, Edward Robb. *A Nation in Torment: The Great American Depression, 1929–1939.* New York: Coward-McCann, 1970.

Enzler, Clarence J. *Some Social Aspects of the Depression (1930–1935).* Washington, DC: The Catholic University of America Press, 1939.

Feinstein, Isidor. "Starving on Relief." *Nation,* February 12, 1936.

"Final Report on the WPA Program." Washington, DC: Work Projects Administration, 1946.

Flexner, Eleanor. "Yes, There Is Starvation in New York City." *Better Times,* April 1932.

*Fortune.* "New York in the Third Winter." January 1932.

———. "'No One Has Starved.'" September 1932.

Frederick, Mrs. Christine. "New Wealth, New Standards of Living and Changed Family Budgets." *Annals of the American Academy of Political and Social Sciences,* September 1924.

———. *Selling Mrs. Consumer.* New York: The Business Bourse, 1929.

Freidel, Frank. *Franklin D. Roosevelt: The Triumph.* Boston: Little, Brown and Company, 1956.

Fritchey, Clayton. "Relief in Ohio." *American Mercury,* May 1940.

Galbraith, John Kenneth. *The Great Crash, 1929.* Boston: Houghton Mifflin, 1955.

Gillett, Lucy H. *Food Primer for the Home.* New York: Bureau of Food Supply, A.I.C.P., 1918.

Gillette, John Morris. *Rural Sociology.* New York: Macmillan Company, 1922.

Goessling, Adeline. *Making the Farm Kitchen Pay.* Springfield, MA: Phelps Pub. Co., 1914.

Goldstein, Carolyn M. *Creating Consumers.* Chapel Hill: University of North Carolina Press, 2012.

Granger, George F., and Lawrence R. Klein. *Emergency Relief in Michigan, 1933–1939.* Lansing, MI: State Emergency Welfare Relief Commission, 1939.

Greenway, John. *American Folksongs of Protest.* New York: Octagon Books, 1970.

Gregory, James N. *American Exodus: The Dust Bowl Migration and Okie Culture in California.* New York: Oxford University Press, 1989.

Gunderson, Gordon W. *The National School Lunch Program: Background and Development.* New York: Nova Science Publishers, 2003.

Haber, William, and Paul L. Stanchfield. *Unemployment and Relief in Michigan.* Lansing, MI: State Emergency Welfare Relief Commission, 1935.

Hackett, Catherine. "'Home Economics,' No Laughing Matter." *Forum and Century,* June 1933.

Hamilton, David E. "Herbert Hoover and the Great Drought of 1930." *Journal of American History,* March 1982.

Harvey, Ray. *Want in the Midst of Plenty: The Genesis of the Food Stamp Plan.* Washington, DC: American Council on Public Affairs, 1941.

Hayes, E. P. *Activities of the President's Emergency Committee for Employment (October 17, 1930–August 19, 1931).* Privately printed, 1936.

Heffernan, Joseph L. "The Hungry City." *The Atlantic*, May 1932.

Henry, Mary, and Day Monroe. "Low Cost Food for Health." *Cornell Bulletin for Homemakers*, June 1932.

Hibben, Sheila. "Food Is to Eat." *Outlook and Independent*, March 20, 1929.

———. *The National Cookbook*. New York: Harper & Brothers, 1932.

Hicks, Floyd W., and C. Roger Lambert. "Food for the Hungry: Federal Food Programs in Arkansas, 1933–1942." *Arkansas Historical Quarterly*, Spring 1978.

Hoff-Wilson, Joan, and Marjorie Lightman, eds. *Without Precedent: The Life and Career of Eleanor Roosevelt*. Bloomington: Indiana University Press, 1984.

Hoover, Herbert. *The Memoirs of Herbert Hoover: The Great Depression, 1929–1941*. New York: Macmillan Company, 1952.

Hoover, Irwin Hood (Ike). *Forty-Two Years in the White House*. Boston: Houghton Mifflin Company, 1934.

Hopkins, Harry. *Relief Needs in New York*. Albany: Temporary Emergency Relief Administration, October 15, 1932.

———. *Spending to Save: The Complete Story of Relief*. New York: W. W. Norton & Co., 1936.

Howard, Donald S. *The WPA and Federal Relief Policy*. New York: Russell Sage Foundation, 1943.

Huzar, Elias. "Federal Unemployment Relief Policies: The First Decade." *Journal of Politics*, August 1940.

Jackson, Gardner. "Unknown Soldiers." *Survey*, August 1, 1932.

Jones, Marian Moser. *The American Red Cross, from Clara Barton to the New Deal*. Baltimore: Johns Hopkins University Press, 2013.

Jordan, Robert. "G.O.P. Budgets for the Hungry." *Nation*, December 23, 1939.

*Journal of Home Economics*. "Adequate Food at Low Cost." February 1932.

———. "Recommended Daily Dietary Allowances." September 1941.

———. "The School Lunch." December 1931.

———. "The School Lunch." January 1938.

*Journal of the American Medical Association*. "Food and Nutrition in the Depression Period." January 2, 1932.

Katz, Michael B. *In the Shadow of the Poorhouse: A Social History of Welfare in America*. New York: Basic Books, 1986.

Kazarian, John. "The Starvation Army." *Nation*, April 26, 1933.

Kerr, Florence. "W.P.A. School Lunch Program." *Journal of Home Economics*, November 1939.

King, Elizabeth Miner. "Dinner-Tables of the Nation." *Harper's Monthly*, December 1, 1918.

Kingseed, Wyatt. "A Promise Denied: The Bonus Expeditionary Force." *American History*, June 2004.

Klein, Nicholas. "Hobo Lingo." *American Speech*, September 1926.

Kline, Ronald R. "Ideology and Social Surveys: Reinterpreting the Effects of 'Laborsaving' Technology on American Farm Women." *Technology and Culture*, April 1997.

Kurlansky, Mark. *Birdseye: The Adventures of a Curious Man*. New York: Doubleday, 2012.

Kusmer, Kenneth L. *Down & Out, On the Road: The Homeless in American History*. New York: Oxford University Press, 2002.

Lange, Dorothea, and Paul Schuster Taylor. *An American Exodus: A Record of Human Erosion in the Thirties*. New Haven: Yale University Press, 1969.

Lash, Joseph P. *Eleanor and Franklin*. New York: W. W. Norton & Company, 1971.

Leitch, I. "The Evolution of Dietary Standards." *Nutrition Abstracts and Reviews*, April 1942.

Le Sueur, Meridel. "Women on the Breadlines." *New Masses*, January 1932.

Leuchtenburg, William E. *Franklin D. Roosevelt and the New Deal, 1932–1940*. New York: Harper & Row, 1963.

———. *Herbert Hoover*. New York: Times Books, 2009.

———. *The Perils of Prosperity, 1914–32*. Chicago: University of Chicago Press, 1958.

Levine, Susan. *School Lunch Politics: The Surprising History of America's Favorite Welfare Program*. Princeton: Princeton University Press, 2008.

*Literary Digest*. "Farm Women Who Count Themselves Blest by Fate." November 13, 1920.

Lohof, Bruce A. "Herbert Hoover, Spokesman of Humane Efficiency: The Mississippi Flood of 1927." *American Quarterly*, Autumn 1970.

Lubell, Samuel, and Walter Everett. "The Breakdown of Relief." *Nation*, August 20, 1938.

Lutes, Della. *The Country Kitchen*. Boston: Little, Brown and Company, 1936.

———. *Home Grown*. Boston: Little, Brown and Company, 1937.

Lynd, Robert S., and Helen Merrell Lynd. *Middletown: A Study in Modern American Culture*. New York: Harcourt, Brace and Company, 1929.

Manchester, William. *The Glory and the Dream: A Narrative History of America, 1932–1972*. Boston: Little, Brown and Company, 1974.

Mason, Mary A. "Nutrition Work Under the Federal Emergency Relief Administration." *Journal of Home Economics*, June–July 1934.

McCollum, Elmer V. *From Kansas Farm Boy to Scientist: The Autobiography of Elmer Verner McCollum*. Lawrence: University of Kansas Press, 1964.

McCollum, Elmer V., and Nina Simonds. *Food, Nutrition and Health*. Baltimore: published by the authors, 1926.

McCormick, Mary G. "The Educational Possibilities of the School Lunch." *Journal of Home Economics*, April 1939.

McWilliams, Carey. *Factories in the Fields: The Story of Migratory Farm Labor in California*. Boston: Little, Brown and Company, 1939.

Melvin, Bruce L. "Rural Life." *American Journal of Sociology*, May 1931.

Mertz, Paul E. *New Deal Policy and Southern Rural Poverty.* Baton Rouge: Louisiana State University Press, 1978.

Milburn, George, ed. *The Hobo's Hornbook.* New York: Ives Washburn, 1930.

Miller, Dorothy Laager. *New York City in the Great Depression: Sheltering the Homeless.* Charleston: Arcadia Publishing, 2009.

Minehan, Thomas. *Boy and Girl Tramps of America.* New York: Farrar and Rinehart, 1934.

Mitchell, Helen S. "The National Nutrition Outlook." *Journal of Home Economics,* October 1941.

Mora, Gilles, and Beverly W. Brannan. *FSA: The American Vision.* New York: Abrams, 2006.

Moran, Rachel Louise. "Consuming Relief: Food Stamps and the New Welfare of the New Deal." *Journal of American History,* March 2011.

Nascher, I. L. *The Wretches of Povertyville.* Chicago: J. J. Lanzit, 1909.

Nash, George H. *The Life of Herbert Hoover: The Humanitarian, 1914–1917.* New York: W. W. Norton & Company, 1988.

*Nation.* "When We Americans Dine: A Symposium on the Great American Dinner." December 26, 1923.

Nesbitt, Henrietta. *The Presidential Cookbook: Feeding the Roosevelts and Their Guests.* Garden City: Doubleday & Company, 1951.

———. *White House Diary.* Garden City, NY: Doubleday & Company, 1948.

Nestle, Marion, and Malden Nesheim. *Why Calories Count: From Science to Politics.* Berkeley: University of California Press, 2012.

New York, N.Y., Department of Public Charities. "Basic Quantity Food Tables To Be Used in Determining the Daily Issue of Food to the Kitchen." July 1912.

New York, N.Y., Department of Public Welfare. *The Men We Lodge.* New York: M. B. Brown Printing & Binding Co., 1915.

New York State Temporary Emergency Relief Administration. *Five Million People, One Billion Dollars.* Albany: Temporary Emergency Relief Administration, June 30, 1937.

———. *Food Allowances.* Albany: Temporary Emergency Relief Administration, August 15, 1932.

Nutrition Bureau. "Food for the Family." New York Association for Improving the Condition of the Poor, 1922.

Ossian, Lisa L. *The Depression Dilemmas of Rural Iowa, 1929–1933.* Columbia: University of Missouri Press, 2011.

Pattison, Mary. *Principles of Domestic Engineering.* New York: Trow Press, 1915.

Pennell, Elizabeth Roberts. "'Eats.'" *North American Review,* March 1922.

Perkins, Frances. *The Roosevelt I Knew.* New York: Viking Press, 1946.

Plunkert, William J. "Public Responsibility for Transients: The Transient Program." *Social Service Review,* March 1, 1934.

Pope, Rowena May. *The Hungry Years: The Story of One Family's Struggle for Survival During the Great Depression*. Circle Pines, MN: Bold Blue Jay Publications, 1982.

Poppendieck, Janet. *Breadlines Knee-Deep in Wheat: Food Assistance in the Great Depression*. Berkeley: University of California Press, 2014.

Reed, Ellery F. *Federal Transient Program: An Evaluative Survey, May to July, 1934*. New York: The Committee on Care of Transient and Homeless, 1934.

*Report of the Activities of the Mayor's Official Committee for the Relief of the Unemployed and Needy of the City of New York, October 31, 1930 to June 30, 1931*. New York: Mayor's Official Committee for the Relief of the Unemployed and Needy of the City of New York, 1931.

"Report of the Country Life Commission." Washington, DC: Government Printing Office, 1909.

Rich, Margaret, ed. *The Administration of Relief in Unemployment Emergencies*. New York: Family Welfare Association of America, 1931.

Robbins, A. "Hunger—1931." *Nation*, February 11, 1931.

Roberts, Warren. "Behind the Cleveland Relief Problem." *Bulletin of the National Tax Association*, March 1, 1940.

Romasco, Albert U. *The Poverty of Abundance*. New York: Oxford University Press, 1965.

Roosevelt, Mrs. Franklin D. *It's Up to the Women*. New York: Frederick A. Stokes Company, 1933.

Rosenman, Samuel I. *Working with Roosevelt*. New York: Da Capo Press, 1972.

Rousseau, Victor. "The Lengthening 'Bread Line.'" *Harper's Weekly*, March 14, 1908.

Salmond, John A. *The Civilian Conservation Corps, 1933–1942: A New Deal Case Study*. Durham, NC: Duke University Press, 1967.

Schlesinger, Arthur M., Jr. *The Politics of Upheaval*. Boston: Houghton Mifflin Company, 1960.

Schneider, David M., and Albert Deutsch. *History of Public Welfare in New York State, 1867–1940*. Chicago: University of Chicago Press, 1938–1941.

Seeber, Frances M. "Eleanor Roosevelt and Women in the New Deal: A Network of Friends." *Presidential Studies Quarterly*, Fall 1990.

Seldes, Gilbert. "Open Your Mouth and Shut Your Eyes." *North American Review*, April 1928.

———. *The Years of the Locust (America, 1929–1932)*. Boston: Little, Brown and Company, 1933.

Shapiro, Laura. "The First Kitchen, Eleanor Roosevelt's Austerity Drive." *New Yorker*, November 22, 2010.

Sherman, Henry C. "Emergency Nutrition." *Child Health Bulletin*, November 1931.

Sherman, Henry C., and Lucy H. Gillett. *The Adequacy and Economy of Some City Dietaries*. New York: Bureau of Food Supply, The New York Association for Improving the Condition of the Poor, 1918.

Sherwood, Robert E. *Roosevelt and Hopkins: An Intimate History.* New York: Harper & Brothers, 1948.

Shideler, James H. "'Flappers and Philosophers,' and Farmers: Rural-Urban Tensions of the Twenties." *Agricultural History,* October 1973.

Shindo, Charles J. *Dust Bowl Migrants in the American Imagination.* Lawrence: University Press of Kansas, 1997.

Smith, Gene. *The Shattered Dream: Herbert Hoover and the Great Depression.* New York: William Morrow & Company, 1970.

*Social Service Review.* "The Disinherited Relief Program." March 1, 1939.

———. "The Food Stamp Plan Comes to Chicago." March 1, 1940.

———. "The Food Stamp Program of Wide Interest." March 1, 1941.

———. "Hunger Is Not Debatable." March 1, 1937.

———. "The Illinois Relief Crisis—And Other Relief Crises, 1938." March 1, 1938.

———. "The 'Liquidation' of the Federal Transient Service." December 1935.

———. "The New York State Temporary Emergency Relief Administration." December 1932.

———. "Three American Poor Relief Documents." June 1929.

Springer, Gertrude. ". . . And What It Has Left Behind." *Survey Midmonthly,* October 1939.

———. "The Federal Bread Line." *Survey Midmonthly,* March 1939.

———. "I Earned It, Didn't I?" *Survey,* April 1936.

———. "Off Again—Relief—On Again." *Survey,* December 1936.

———. "Ragged White Collars." *Survey,* November 15, 1931.

———. "Relief in November 1939." *Survey Midmonthly,* November 1938.

———. "Where Is the Money Coming From?" *Survey,* October 15, 1931.

Starr, Kathy. *The Soul of Southern Cooking.* Jackson: University Press of Mississippi, 1989.

Steinbeck, John. "Dubious Battle in California." *Nation,* September 12, 1936.

———. *Their Blood Is Strong.* San Francisco: Simon J. Lubin Society of California, 1938.

Stiebeling, Hazel K. *Food Budgets for Nutrition and Production Programs.* Department of Agriculture Miscellaneous Publication No. 183, Washington, DC: Government Printing Office, December 1933.

Stiebeling, Hazel K., and Miriam Birdseye. *Adequate Diets for Families with Limited Incomes.* U.S. Department of Agriculture, Miscellaneous Publications No. 113, Washington, DC: Government Printing Office, April 1931.

*Survey.* "New Faces on the Bowery." April 1, 1930.

———. "The Relief State of the Nation." January 1936.

Sutherland, Edwin H., and Harvey J. Locke. *Twenty Thousand Homeless Men: A Study of Unemployed Men in the Chicago Shelters.* Chicago: J. B. Lippincott Company, 1936.

Taylor, Carl. "The Rise of the Rural Problem." *Journal of Social Forces,* November 1923.

Taylor, Carl C., et al. "Disadvantaged Classes in American Agriculture." Social Research Report no. VIII. Washington, DC: United States Department of Agriculture, April 1938.

Taylor, Lea D. "Decent Standards of Relief." *Survey*, May 15, 1932.

Taylor, Paul S., and Tom Vasey. "Drought Refugee and Labor Migration to California, June–December 1935." *Monthly Labor Review*, February 1936.

Terrill, Tom E., and Jerrold Hirsch, eds. *Such as Us: Southern Voices of the Thirties*. Chapel Hill: University of North Carolina Press, 1978.

*Transients in California*. Sacramento: State Relief Administration of California, 1936.

Trattner, Walter I. *From Poor Law to Welfare State: A History of Social Welfare in America*, 6th ed. New York: The Free Press, 1999.

United States Children's Bureau. *Emergency Food Relief and Child Health*. Washington, DC: Government Printing Office, 1931.

———. *Family Food Budgets for the Use of Relief Agencies*. Washington, DC: Government Printing Office, 1932.

United States Department of Agriculture. *Social and Labor Needs of Farm Women*. Washington, DC: Government Printing Office, 1915.

Vance, Rupert B. *Human Factors in Cotton Culture: A Study in the Social Geography of the American South*. Chapel Hill: University of North Carolina Press, 1929.

Ward, Florence E. "The Farm Woman's Problems." *Journal of Home Economics*, October 1920.

Wasserman, Suzanne. "'Our Alien Neighbors': Coping with the Depression on the Lower East Side." *American Jewish History*, June 1, 2000.

Waters, W. W. *B.E.F.: The Whole Story of the Bonus Army*. New York: The John Day Company, 1933.

Watkins, Lucy Rodgers, ed. *A Generation Speaks: Voices of the Great Depression*. Chapel Hill: Chapel Hill Press, 2000.

Westfall, Martha, and Josephine M. Adams. "Emergency Lunches in New York City." *Practical Home Economics*, March 1932.

Wharton, Don. "The Federal Food-Stamp Plan." *American Mercury*, April 1940.

Whisenhunt, Donald W. "The Great Depression in Kentucky: The Early Years." *Register of the Kentucky Historical Society*, January 1969.

Williams, James Mickel. *Human Aspects of Unemployment and Relief*. Chapel Hill: University of North Carolina Press, 1933.

Wilson, Robert S., and Dorothy B. de la Pole. *Group Treatment for Transients*. New York: National Association for Travelers Aid and Transient Service, 1935.

Woodruff, Nan. *As Rare as Rain: Federal Relief in the Great Southern Drought of 1930–31*. Urbana: University of Illinois Press, 1985.

Woodward, Ellen S. "The Works Progress Administration School Lunch Project." *Journal of Home Economics*, November 1936.

Workless [pseud.]. "I'm Tired of Beans." *Nation*, January 28, 1931.

Wunder, John R., et al., eds. *Americans View Their Dust Bowl Experience.* Niwot: University Press of Colorado, 1999.

Zimmerman, Julie N. *Opening Windows onto Hidden Lives: Women, Country Life, and Early Rural Sociological Research.* University Park: Pennsylvania State University Press, 2010.

Zinn, Howard, ed. *New Deal Thought.* Indianapolis: Bobbs-Merrill Company, Inc., 1966.

# Index

Entries in *italics* refer to illustrations.

## About the Authors

JANE ZIEGELMAN is the author of the widely acclaimed *97 Orchard: An Edible History of Five Immigrant Families in One New York Tenement*, a finalist for an IACP award, and which is currently being made into a PBS documentary. Jane curates food-themed events for the Tenement Museum. Jane has lectured on food history for cultural institutions around the country and has appeared in food documentaries such as *Deli Man* and *Appetite City*. She lives in Brooklyn with her husband—and writing partner—Andrew Coe, and their two boys.

ANDREW COE is a writer and independent scholar specializing in culinary history. His groundbreaking *Chop Suey: A Cultural History of Chinese Food in the United States* was a finalist for a James Beard Award and named one of the best food books of the year by the *Financial Times*. He has written books, articles, and blog posts on everything from the ancient history of foie gras to the secret criminal past of chocolate egg creams to where to buy the tastiest bread in New York City. He has appeared in documentaries such as the National Geographic Channel's *Eat: The Story of Food* and *The Search for General Tso*. He lives in Brooklyn with wife and coauthor, Jane Ziegelman. They have two children.